Transition Assessment

Transition Assessment

Wise Practices for Quality Lives

by

Caren L. Sax, Ed.D.
San Diego State University

and

Colleen A. Thoma, Ph.D.
University of Nevada—Las Vegas

with invited contributors

Foreword by Jeffrey Strully, M.S.

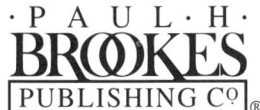

Baltimore • London • Toronto • Sydney

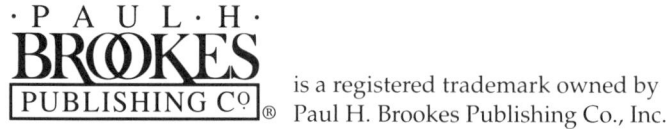 is a registered trademark owned by Paul H. Brookes Publishing Co., Inc.

Paul H. Brookes Publishing Co.
Post Office Box 10624
Baltimore, Maryland 21285-0624

www.brookespublishing.com

Copyright © 2002 by Paul H. Brookes Publishing Co., Inc.
All rights reserved.

Typeset by Integrated Publishing Solutions, Grand Rapids, Michigan.
Manufactured in the United States of America by
Sheridan Books, Fredericksburg, Virginia.

Most cases described in this book are composites based on the authors' actual experiences. In these instances, individuals' names have been changed and identifying details have been altered to protect confidentiality. Real names and stories are used by permission.

Library of Congress Cataloging-in-Publication Data

Transition assessment: wise practices for quality lives / by Caren L. Sax
    and Colleen A. Thoma.
        p.   cm.
    Includes bibliographical references and index.
    ISBN 1-55766-570-2
    1. Handicapped—Functional assessment.   I. Sax, Caren L.   II. Thoma, Colleen A.
    RM930.8 .T73   2002
    616.85′8803—dc21   2001043617

British Library Cataloguing in Publication data are available from the British Library.

Contents

About the Authors ... vii
About the Contributors ... ix
Foreword   *Jeffrey Strully* ... xiii
To Our Readers ... xvii
Acknowledgments ... xix

1   For Whom the Test Is Scored:
Assessments, the School Experience, and More
Douglas Fisher and Caren L. Sax ... 1

2   Person-Centered Planning: More than a Strategy
Caren L. Sax ... 13

3   Self-Determined Assessment:
Critical Components for Transition Planning
Michael L. Wehmeyer ... 25

4   The Three C's of Family Involvement:
Things I Wish I Had Known
Barbara Buswell and Caren L. Sax ... 39

5   Informal Assessment Procedures
Carolyn Hughes and Erik W. Carter ... 51

6   Measuring What's Important: Using Alternative Assessments
Colleen A. Thoma and Mary Held ... 71

7   Assessing Individual Needs for Assistive Technology
Gerald Craddock and Marcia J. Scherer ... 87

8   Vocational and Career Assessment
Patricia Rogan, Teresa A. Grossi, and Roberta Gajewski ... 103

9   Transition Service Integration Model: Ensuring that the
Last Day of School Is No Different from the Day After
*Nicholas J. Certo, Caren L. Sax, Ian Pumpian, Denise Mautz,
Kimberly A. Smalley, Holly A. Wade, and David A. Noyes* ... 119

10   Putting Transition Plans into Action:
"I Don't Want to Count Money at Home Anymore!"
Caren L. Sax and Colleen A. Thoma ... 133

Coda   The Watergivers: A History of a Helping Profession
Scot Danforth ... 141

Index ... 147

About the Authors

Caren L. Sax, Ed.D., Assistant Professor, Department of Administration, Rehabilitation, and Postsecondary Education, San Diego State University, 3590 Camino del Rio North, San Diego, California 92108

Dr. Sax is Assistant Professor in San Diego State University's rehabilitation counseling graduate program. She also coordinates the Certificate of Rehabilitation Technology with the College of Engineering and the Pupil Personnel Services credential with the Department of Counseling and School Psychology. She has taught courses in assistive technology, transition, special education, and rehabilitation, both on campus and via distance education. Through funding from federal and state grant projects, she has directed research, demonstration, and training projects related to the applications of assistive technology, systems change efforts for school-to-adult life transition services for students with disabilities, and continuing education opportunities for community rehabilitation personnel. Dr. Sax has written extensively and presents at conferences, seminars, and symposia held locally, statewide, nationally, and internationally.

Colleen A. Thoma, Ph.D., Assistant Professor, College of Education, Department of Special Education, University of Nevada–Las Vegas, 4505 South Maryland Parkway, Box 453014, Las Vegas, Nevada 89154

Dr. Thoma coordinates the graduate programs in teaching students with severe disabilities and the program for transition planning at the University of Nevada–Las Vegas. She has taught courses on transition planning, augmentative and alternative communication, curriculum development, assessment, and the medical aspects of disabilities. Through grant-funded projects, she has conducted research in the areas of teacher education, alternative assessment, positive behavior supports, and self-determination in transition planning. Dr. Thoma has published articles and made presentations on self-determined transition planning, alternative assessment in transition planning, and a multicultural perspective of self-determination.

About the Contributors

Barbara Buswell, M.A., is Executive Director of the PEAK Parent Center, a former high school English teacher, and the parent of three children (ages 18, 22, and 23). Her middle son, Wilson, has physical and communication challenges and used intensive supports and resources to attend his neighborhood school and general education classrooms. Ms. Buswell has a master's degree in inclusive educational reform and is interested in the intersection of general and special education as well as the transition from quality schooling to an inclusive life. Her family has been living the experiences that this book addresses.

Erik W. Carter, M.S., is a research assistant with the Department of Special Education at Vanderbilt University. Mr. Carter previously worked as a transition teacher in San Antonio, Texas. He is co-author of *The Transition Handbook: Strategies High School Teachers Use that Work!* (with Carolyn Hughes, Paul H. Brookes Publishing Co., 2000) and has authored manuscripts in the areas of transition and peer interactions. Mr. Carter received a master's degree in special education in 1998 from Vanderbilt University, where he currently is pursuing a doctoral degree in special education.

Nicholas J. Certo, Ph.D., Professor of Special Education at San Francisco State University, received his doctoral degree from the Department of Behavioral Disorders at the University of Wisconsin in 1976. He is among the first professionals in the United States to have demonstrated that individuals with significant support needs could learn to function and work in integrated community settings and is credited with editing the first textbook in his subspecialty area, severe disabilities. Prior to his current position, he was employed as a project officer in the U.S. Bureau of Education for the Handicapped, as an Executive Assistant to the Assistant Secretary for Planning and Evaluation in the U.S. Department of Health and Human Services, and as an Assistant Professor in the Department of Special Education at the University of Maryland at College Park. He has published widely on the subject of transition to work and community living for youth with significant support needs and has a long and consistent record of receiving federal funding to support the development of innovative approaches to transition.

Gerald Craddock, BEng, M.S.E.E, has worked in the area of technology and disability since 1983. He has been the manager of the client technical services (CTS) department of the Central Remedial Clinic (CRC) in Dublin, Ireland, since 1991. He works with a staff of 18 people who have backgrounds in many disciplines, from paramedical to technical, to social. The CRC is a nonresidential center that provides assessment and therapy services to children and adults with physical and multiple disabilities. Mr. Craddock has implemented a number of Irish and European projects in the advancement of assistive technology and in particular striving to include people with disabilities as the service providers in this area. He is presently working on a doctorate in the area of assistive technology and students with disabilities.

About the Contributors

Scot Danforth, Ph.D., Associate Professor of Education at the University of Missouri–St. Louis, is the author of numerous articles examining the social and political construction of disability in society and schools. He is co-founder of the Disability Studies in Education Special Interest Group of the American Educational Research Association and co-editor of the journal *Disability, Culture, and Education.*

Douglas Fisher, Ph.D., Associate Professor of Teacher Education at San Diego State University, serves as the Director of Professional Development for the City Heights Educational Pilot. This pilot is a partnership between San Diego State University and an elementary, middle, and high school, focused on improving the educational experiences for 5,000 public school children in three inner city schools and improving the likelihood that these students attend college. In addition, Dr. Fisher is a teacher, teacher educator, and writer. His writing has appeared in *The California Reader*, *Remedial and Special Education*, and the *Journal of Adolescent and Adult Literacy*. He is the co-author of four books focused on curriculum development and modification.

Roberta Gajewski, M.S., Visiting Lecturer in the School of Education at Indiana University–Purdue University, Indianapolis, has 33 years of experience as an educator and 26 years of personal experience as the mother of a daughter with a disability. Ms. Gajewski served as a founding member of a parent support goup in Indianapolis and has been active in local and state advisory groups. She was a transition specialist, co-directed TIES (Transition Integrated Employment Services), authored a series of booklets on transition issues, and most recently contributed to *Personnel Preparation in Disability and Community Life* by Julie Ann Racino (Charles C. Thomas, 2000). She received an education award in Indiana for her work in transition and has been an advocate for individuals with disabilities through the Indiana Resource Center for Families with Special Needs. She and her daughter have presented at local, state, and national conferences.

Teresa A. Grossi, Ph.D., Director of the Center on Community Living and Careers at the Indiana Institute on Disability and Community, has extensive background in education and employment for individuals with disabilities. She has worked in North Carolina and Ohio as a community-based instructor, transition coordinator, and job coach and managed a vocational training program and a supported employment agency. Prior to working in Indiana, Dr. Grossi directed Ohio's systems change grant in supported employment and co-chaired the cross-training team for the Transition from School to Adult Life systems change grant. Dr. Grossi conducts research, consultation, training, and technical assistance on supported employment and community supports for individuals with severe disabilities. Specifically, her research focuses on systems change issues and strategies to facilitate the integration and employment opportunities for individuals with disabilities.

Mary Held, M.S., C.R.C., doctoral candidate at Indiana University, is completing her dissertation on teacher implementation of self-determination strategies in a secondary classroom, focused primarily on the transition planning and assessment process. She has conducted research in the areas of conversion from segregated workshops to community-based employment, transition planning, and student empowerment. She is teaching at Indiana University–Purdue University, Indianapolis.

Carolyn Hughes, Ph.D, Associate Professor in the Department of Special Education at Vanderbilt University, serves as Project Director of the federally funded Metropolitan Nashville Peer Buddy Program. She teaches, researches, and publishes in the areas of self-instruction and self-determination, transition from school to adult life, and social interaction and social inclusion of high school students. Dr. Hughes co-authored *The Transition Handbook: Strategies High School Teachers Use that Work!* (with Erik W. Carter, Paul H. Brookes Publishing Co., 2000).

Denise Mautz, M.A., is a doctoral degree candidate studying special education at the University of California–Berkeley and San Francisco State University. Ms. Mautz co-directed the first completely community-based integrated work and community inclusion agency in one Bay Area county, while earning her master of arts degree in vocational special education at San Francisco State University. She is currently focusing on policy and practice related to transition and adult services, integrated adult service staff management systems, progressive job development for people labeled unemployable, and state-of-the-art adult service delivery.

David A. Noyes , M.S., is a vocational rehabilitation counselor with the state of California. He has a master's degree in rehabilitation counseling and is completing his doctoral dissertation at the University of San Diego. Mr. Noyes specializes in supported employment and, as a Program Specialist with the Interwork Institute at San Diego State University, coordinates the implementation and replication of the Point of Transition Service Integration model.

Ian Pumpian, Ph.D., Professor of Education Leadership at San Diego State University, also serves as Executive Director of the City Heights Educational Pilot—a cooperative agreement with three San Diego City schools, the San Diego Education Association, San Diego State University, and Price Charities focused on improving student achievement in urban schools. Dr. Pumpian designed the Supported Employment and Transition Services Specialist Certificate at San Diego State University and has published in the area of transition, employment, and inclusive communities for people with significant disabilities.

Patricia Rogan, Ph.D., Associate Professor at Indiana University, teaches in the area of special education and is a research associate at the Indiana Institute on Disability and Community, Indiana's University Center for Excellence on Disabilities. She prepares school and adult service personnel, provides training and technical assistance within Indiana and nationally, and conducts research and writing related to transition and employment.

Marcia J. Scherer, Ph.D., M.P.H., is the author of *Living in the State of Stuck: How Assistive Technology Impacts the Lives of People with Disabilities* (Brookline, 2000) and co-editor of *Evaluating, Selecting, and Using Appropriate Assistive Technology* (Aspen Publishers, 1996) and *Psychological Assessment in Medical Rehabilitation* (with Cushman, American Psychological Association, 1995). Dr. Scherer is on the editorial boards of *Disability and Rehabilitation* and *Assistive Technology*. She is a Fellow of the American Psychological Association, Division of Rehabilitation Psychology, as well as in the Division of Applied Experimental and Engineering Psychology. In addition to directing the Institute for Matching Person and Technology, Dr. Scherer is Senior Research Associate at the International Center for Hearing and Speech Research (University of Rochester and Rochester Institute of Technology) and Associate Professor of Physical Medicine and Rehabilitation at the University of Rochester Medical Center.

Kimberly A. Smalley, Ph.D., is the Mental Retardation/Developmental Disabilities Behavior Specialist at the Hawaii State Department of Health, Children and Adolescent Mental Health Division. She is available statewide to children and their teams to collaboratively increase replacement behaviors and create a better quality of life. She provides training and support to promote positive behavioral supports as a statewide agenda. Prior to her current position, she was employed as a behavioral consultant in the San Francisco Bay area, where she served children and families with significant needs and behavior challenges through the local school districts, Department of Developmental Disabilities, vocational rehabilitation, and service providers. She has demonstrated a long history of advocacy and support for human rights. She presents nationally and locally to promote the use of child-centered, self-determined, positive behavioral support plans that enhance skill development and quality of life.

Holly A. Wade, M.A., has more than 12 years experience in the area of transition from school to work and has considerable expertise in self-advocacy and sexuality for individuals with significant disabilities. She has taught university courses at San Jose State University and San Francisco State University and worked in public school settings. Ms. Wade has provided many in-services and has presented at conferences on sexuality and social relationships among individuals with disabilities. Ms. Wade also is a student in the joint doctoral program in special education between San Francisco State University and the University of California–Berkeley.

Michael L. Wehmeyer, Ph.D., Associate Professor of Special Education, also serves as the Assistant Director of the Beach Center on Disability, University of Kansas. He directs multiple federally funded projects to conduct research on and develop methods and materials to promote the self-determination of children, youth, and adults with cognitive and developmental disabilities. He has authored more than 80 articles or book chapters. In addition, he has authored or edited 10 books on self-determination, student involvement, transition, and assistive technology.

Foreword

My son, Alex, and his friend, Robin, left for an extended trip to Europe as soon as they finished high school. They spent several months traveling around Europe enjoying life in foreign countries. Alex and Robin traveled mostly by train, stayed at youth hostels, and found ways to eat cheaply, mostly existing on cheese, bread, and wine. They enjoyed the variety and novelty of traveling in different countries but spent most of their time in Germany, France, England, and Ireland. Whether camping on the beach in Nice in the winter or visiting sites in England where Jack the Ripper killed his victims, the adventurers explored places off the beaten track. Alex and Robin met lots of local people who welcomed them to their countries and, at times, into their homes. They showed the young Americans around their countries, developing friendships that have lasted many years after the journey ended. Alex and Robin visited traditional places as well and, of course, had a taste of the nightlife that each country offered.

Upon returning home, Alex and Robin decided to travel through the states. By May, they wanted to watch the Kentucky Derby from the infield and then go on to Indiana to cheer from the bleachers at the Indianapolis 500. They camped in Oregon, whale watched in Washington, hiked through the Grand Canyon, and experienced life on the Boston Common. My son and his friend wanted to see lots of different things throughout our country and to continue to just enjoy life for a while.

Ultimately, Alex went on to work for a large fast-food restaurant for several years. He lived with several different roommates, attended community college to become an auto body mechanic, and continued to travel. Several years later, he moved into the mountains outside of Santa Cruz, California, and currently lives in a wonderful house with large trees in the front yard. The house is located in a great neighborhood. Alex works part time as a laborer doing construction work. He has lots of friends and other connections in the community. He enjoys being a regular at an English pub in Boulder Creek and going to summer concerts on the beach in Santa Cruz. Life is good; it is filled with exciting moments amidst the normal routines and rhythms.

Oh, by the way, Alex has Down syndrome!

Alex truly experienced life during the transition from school to adulthood. Unfortunately, when Alex graduated, this was the exception and not the rule. People with developmental disabilities typically did not have the same opportunities as their peers without disabilities to experience a wide variety of options after graduating high school as they tried to figure out what they wanted to be when they grew up. For most people with developmental disabilities, transition planning usually resulted in placement in a sheltered workshop, enclave, or mobile crew, while living at home with parents or maybe moving into a group home or intermediate care facility for people with mental retardation. If these people were very, very lucky, perhaps someone mentioned supported employment and supported living, but this situation did not occur very often, especially if their needs were viewed as "more intensive."

Assessment tools and strategies did not really look at creative and thoughtful ways to support individuals, especially people with more intense support needs, to have good lives. Most of these assessment tools and strategies tended to blame people with disabilities for not achieving quality lives. It was the individual's fault. If students with disabilities would only learn, get their behaviors under control, and stop causing problems, then they would be able to earn their way to a good life. We blamed the victims for why their lives were not better. We used "official protocol" that allowed us to reject people from thinking creatively and pursuing things that were important to them. We were able to stand behind our professionalism to confidently tell people why they would never accomplish a certain goal or achieve a desired outcome. It was a safe place for many professionals to be.

Because many people, including parents and professionals, relegated people with disabilities to low status, low expectations became a self-fulfilling prophecy. People with disabilities too often led marginal, miserable lives. They were rejected from "mainstream" life in the community because of their disabilities. Because of these attitudes, dreaming about desirable futures did not come easily for many families who have sons and daughters with significant disabilities. The dreams of people with disabilities and their families were squashed, or at least stifled, by far too many professionals in the name of adhering to the system. Seeing people with disabilities as contributing, valued members of our community was not even on the radar screen.

When I first read the proposal for this book, I found it difficult to provide a response to the outline without knowing who would be writing the chapters. Even though I understood the need for a blind review, I thought it was important to know who the authors were, what they believed, and what they have done in their lives. I did not want to support some sort of theoretical exercise. People use words, but you are never sure if what they mean is what you think the word means. The word *assessment* is one that always makes me suspicious. Too often, assessment instruments have turned out to be professional strategies to prevent people with significant disabilities from living, playing, working, and having friends in the community. Predicting whether this type of book would be based on work in the real world or on a concept of what that real world might be was difficult without knowing the values and philosophies of the authors.

But I discovered that this book attempts to break out of the traditional way of thinking that most stakeholders get stuck in when involved with transition planning. It attempts to get people out of stereotyped boxes when thinking about possibilities for the future. It further attempts to help the reader think creatively about all of the opportunities available to people as they take their unique personal journeys through adult life. Whether it is going to work, starting a business, going to college, traveling, buying a home of their own, or getting married, it doesn't really matter. What does matter is that all of these options, not just some of them, should be both open and actively available to all people. Availability should not be based on the perceived skills and competencies that an individual might possess or that a "test" may indicate. What we need to see is for *all* people to have *all* options available to them as they move forward with their personal journeys.

This book attempts to help all of the stakeholders who are surrounding the person with a disability to think more creatively about possibilities. It also provides an opportunity for families, consumers, and those involved with transition planning to think of new and different options. The questions, "What do you want to do with your life, and how can we support you?" are well worth asking people with disabilities and their families. Asking these questions forces us to learn to listen to people more deeply and to honor and respect their dreams. It also helps us to understand the importance of providing support and assistance to people so that they can move closer to living out their dreams. It further urges us to learn ways to figure out how to plan and design supports so that people can enjoy a valued and wonderful life in the community. There are no simple gimmicks or short cuts to learning to listen, getting to know people, and figuring out what people want to do with their lives. Although there are no easy answers, there are tools that can assist. There are also strategies to help people figure out the transition needs of an individual.

Times are indeed changing. People with all levels of disabilities are taking their rightful place in society as contributing and exciting members. It is neither easy nor simple. Things do not necessarily work out perfectly the first time; however, we are seeing a change in the way people with disabilities experience life in the community. This book will assist all stakeholders involved in transition planning to better understand people with disabilities and how to support them as they transition to a new exciting adventure in their lives. Equally important will be the change in behaviors of these stakeholders to enable people with disabilities to truly experience the transition from teenager to adult with excitement and passion.

The way to think about transition is to bring people together, listen to their dreams, figure out ways for them to work on their dreams, utilize resources in ways that make sense, try and fail, then regroup and try again. Most people with more intensive support needs will only really succeed if we listen to them and travel with them on their personal journeys. Assessment strategies can be used to eliminate, reduce, or minimize people's dreams or, as presented in this book, assessment strategies can be wise, thoughtful, supportive, and dynamic. Let us begin the journey . . .

Jeffrey Strully, M.S.
Executive Director
Jay Nolan Community Services
Mission Hills, California

To Our Readers

We all experience transitions throughout our lives. This book focuses on the transitions of young adults with disabilities who are exiting the school system and entering adult life. After countless discussions with families and professionals, we created this book as a tool for young adults with disabilities who are beginning the transition process, as well as for those whose job or life-role places them in a supporting role (e.g., family, school personnel, friends, adult agency staff). We know that for many, assessments have become something to avoid or at best live through. They have been used to justify segregated educational placements, highlight disabilities as opposed to abilities, and limit future possibilities. In the last few years, assessment and testing have acquired even more emphasis and, with that, more negative connotations. In the name of standards and accountability, testing (or assessment) has further limited the ability of many high school students with disabilities to become college students. Not because of a failure on their part to learn, but because of a failure to demonstrate what they know through a paper and pencil test. So, why would we write a book on transition assessment?

Primarily, we wanted to increase awareness. We also wanted to provide user-friendly strategies and examples of students in transition implementing these strategies. We wanted more people to know that there are effective assessment approaches and procedures that can provide essential information for making wise choices about the future. Wise choices depend on recording and relaying information about what a student can do, what he or she enjoys doing, and what preferences he or she has for an adult lifestyle. Yet, many professionals tend to rely on traditional, standardized assessment procedures or are required to use these formal tools by the systems in which they work. Formal tools can be useful in determining eligibility for services but have limited usefulness for determining the supports to be addressed.

In this era of standardized testing, we wrote this book as a reminder about the true spirit and promise of assessment—taking the time to get acquainted with people and to begin to understand who they are and what they want to do. While wise practices in assessment take time, they reap abundant information for making choices and identifying necessary supports so that student preferences for an adult lifestyle become a reality. We hope that the information in this book will provide a variety of transition assessment strategies that can help in making wise decisions about adult life. Having been through the process with friends and family, we believe that individualizing the assessment process is the best way to meet the needs of students and their families who are facing this major change in their lives.

Acknowledgments

Our first venture together as co-authors was successful mainly due to the personal commitment and passion that we each have for this topic. Securing support from our colleagues and families gave us the motivation to "transition" from a good idea to a reality—one that would not likely have happened without their patience and belief in us and in the project.

We would first like to acknowledge Lisa Benson, our acquisitions editor at Brookes Publishing Co., who trusted our talent and our ability to put the right information into words. She and her staff guided us through the publication process with finesse and respect. The colleagues we contacted to write chapters possessed values that were consistent with the holistic and person-centered philosophy that we used as the foundation of this book. Each of the chapter authors had a unique perspective to add to the mix, representing families, public schools, universities, and community agencies, both in the United States of America and in Ireland. Their interest and willingness to share their experience and expertise have made this book useful to students and families facing the transition from school to adult life as well as to the professionals who can make this challenging period more seamless.

A special acknowledgment goes to Doug Fisher, who urged us to take on this endeavor and who helped us when we got stuck. His professional and personal generosity is always given freely and unequivocally.

Finally, we would like to thank our families—Chris, Michael, and Christopher—who gave up family time once again and waited patiently as we rushed to meet another deadline and finished one more set of edits. They made us promise that we would take some time off as soon as this was completed!

To Julie, Peyton, and Stephen
—C.L.S.

To Beth, Katie, and Santa
—C.A.T.

and all of the other students and families who have taught us about collaboration, relationships, and transition

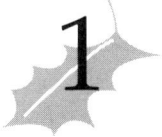

For Whom the Test Is Scored

Assessments, the School Experience, and More

Douglas Fisher and Caren L. Sax

PUSHING THE LIMITS FOR JOSHUA'S FUTURE

The telephone rings, and I answer. "Hello?" The voice on the other end quietly asks, "How do I get my kid into college?" My initial response is, "Did your son or daughter apply?" There is a pause, and then the answer, "No, he has a disability, and I'm not sure how he'll do in college, but he really wants to go." I have to ask the next question, "Has he been in regular high school classes? Does he know about the general education curriculum?" Thankfully, she answers, "Yes! And he's been volunteering in a music store. Joshua loves music and really wants to learn more about it at college." I can hardly contain my excitement, and I say, "Great, get an application and get him into school! He'll need an appointment with someone in student services who can coordinate the supports, accommodations, and modifications he'll need to be successful." I'm thinking smugly to myself, "No problem—we'll get him into college easily."

Then, with tears, she drops the bomb: "The funding agency says that their assessments show that he can't work and that college wouldn't benefit him. I can't afford for him to attend college without financial help. I'm a single mom with other kids to feed." Hiding my own disappointment, I ask, "What assessments did they do?" His mom tells me that she can't remember. I ask if someone came to the school, work, or home to conduct the assessments. She says no, they reviewed his file and said that he didn't qualify. I

Previous versions of parts of this chapter have appeared in Fisher, D., & Sax, C. (1999). Noticing differences between secondary and postsecondary education: Extending Agran, Snow, and Swaner's discussion. *The Journal of The Association for Persons with Severe Handicaps, 24,* 303–305. Used with permission from The Association for Persons with Severe Handicaps.

try to explain that those aren't assessments, they are judgments. I tell her that I'd be happy to meet her son and talk with the two of them about options. I also tell her that we're getting started a little late and that my understanding of assessments suggests that they be used to provide instructional guidance, rally support, and ensure funding. We agree to meet for coffee and talk further.

When I meet Joshua, I know that he is a great candidate for college and paid employment. I am pleased that I have an assessment repertoire that allows me to understand Joshua and his unique strengths. I am also pleased that his general and special education teachers in middle school and high school have maintained a portfolio of "successful strategies" and support plans over the years . . . our work is ready to begin!

WHAT IS ASSESSMENT?

The term *assessment* comes from the Latin word *assidere,* which literally means "to sit with." It seems that this is a great place to start. Individuals with significant disabilities need someone to sit with, someone who will get to know them well and who will help them organize information about their lives—both past history and future dreams—in a respectful and meaningful way. This book provides a plethora of examples and ways in which assessments can be used to improve the quality of life outcomes that people with significant disabilities experience; however, before engaging in a meaningful conversation about assessments, the environments and systems in which people with significant disabilities are educated need to be examined. These assessments will be influenced in part by the values of the support staff, the quality of the environments to which individuals have access, and the willingness of others to engage in activities that are meaningful. This chapter provides an overview of the educational systems for individuals with significant disabilities and the difference between secondary and postsecondary education. It concludes with a set of questions about assessment strategies. These questions guide the formation of wise practices necessary for creating quality lives.

OVERVIEW OF EDUCATIONAL OPPORTUNITIES

Adult life for most people is a unique balance of work, home, recreation, and learning. Where people spend time, what they spend time doing, and with whom they establish relationships seem to best reflect their circumstances, plans, accomplishments, shortcomings, and qualities of life. Most of adult life is a result of an interest in establishing bonds, relationships, and experiences with others. These relationships affect access, opportunity, stability, and change. Physical, emotional, social, and intellectual well-being are directly related to the *where, what,* and *who* in people's lives. This rich combination of choice, access, activity, balance, and relationships is what people typically mean by quality of life.

Clearly, early experience, including education, strongly influences the quality of one's adult life (Feinberg & Soltis, 1992; Oakes & Lipton, 1990). There is little debate regarding a school's responsibility to prepare its learners for the future. Business leaders have become increasingly critical of schools as they see inadequately educated young people entering the workforce (Wilson & Daviss, 1994). These business leaders, as well as parents and community members, expect graduates who can solve problems, think critically, work on a team, and make clear judgments. Schools are preparatory in nature, and communities are beginning to hold them responsible for preparing youngsters for adult life (U.S. Department of Education, 1994b).

Schools are being held accountable not only for the outcomes of typical students, but for those of students with disabilities as well. One body of literature related to these criteria of ultimate functioning evaluates the service delivery system in terms of innovation, comprehensiveness, person-centered focus, and effect on the student's quality of life (Brown, 1991; Calculator & Jorgensen, 1994; Stainback, Stainback, & Forest, 1989). The expectation is that education should contribute to the preparation that all U.S. citizens need to fully and meaningfully participate in public life. This right is deeply embedded in U.S. law and heritage; it is an inalienable right (Gilhool, 1976). It is the responsibility of educators to help ensure that all U.S. citizens, regardless of their abilities, are afforded an equal opportunity to actively participate in all community activities, events, and opportunities. Outcome-based questions have become a standard for evaluating the effectiveness of education (i.e., Has the school system done its job in preparing students with disabilities for adult lives, which involve work, home, and social environments?).

DO SCHOOL SYSTEMS PREPARE STUDENTS WITH DISABILITIES FOR WORK AND ADULT LIFE?

Data from the National Longitudinal Transition Study of Special Education Students (Wagner, 1993), among other studies (e.g., Aune, 1991; Malakpa, 1994; Mithaug, Moriuchi, & Fanning, 1985), have documented poor postschool outcomes for students with disabilities. In addition to high dropout rates (58%), these students often exit into low-wage jobs, have higher arrest records (44%), and are unemployed in vast numbers (60%). After more than 20 years of specific federal support through the Education for All Handicapped Children Act of 1975 (PL 94-142), and its current reauthorization, the Individuals with Disabilities Education Act (IDEA) Amendments of 1997 (PL 105-17), fewer than half of the students receiving special education services graduate with a diploma (U.S. Department of Education, 1993). According to the National Longitudinal Transition Study, only 20% of young adults with disabilities are independent in the domains of work, residential activities, and social activities by the time they have been out of school for 3–5 years. Fewer than 30% of students classified as having mild speech-language impairments or mild learning disabilities obtained independence in all three of these domains (U.S. Department of Education, 1993). These students, assured by PL 94-142 and its subsequent amendments of an appropriate education until completion of high school or age 21, are opting instead to abandon those mandated services (Zigmond & Thornton, 1985). Wehlage and Rutter (1986) argued that it is the school, and not the student, that must change if appreciable improvements are to be made.

The outcomes for students with severe disabilities have been even less impressive (Braddock & Mitchell, 1992; Cole & Meyer, 1991; Evans & Scotti, 1989). These students have been described in a variety of ways, many of which convey hopelessness and despair. These historical definitions include such terms as *extremely debilitating, inflexibly incapacitated,* and *uncompromisingly crippled* (McDonnell, Hardman, McDonnell, & Kiefer-O'Donnell, 1995, p. 3). Others have described students with severe disabilities based on a discrepancy from what is considered to be typically developing. Justen proposed such a definition:

> The "severely handicapped" refers to those individuals age 21 and younger who are functioning at a general development level of half or less than the level which would be expected on the basis of chronological age and who manifest learning and/or behavior problems of such magnitude and significance that they require extensive structure in learning situations if their education needs are to be well served. (1976, p. 5)

A more modern definition that continues to be used is based on the instructional needs of the student and was offered by Meyer, Peck, and Brown:

> These people include individuals of all ages who require extensive ongoing support in more than one major life activity in order to participate in inclusive community environments and to enjoy a quality of life that is available to citizens with fewer or more disabilities. Support may be required for life activities such as mobility, communication, self-care, and learning as necessary for independent living, employment, and self-sufficiency. (1991, p. 19)

It is clear that students with significant disabilities require extensive supports and challenge the educational system's ability to provide an appropriate education.

WHAT LAWS AFFECT OUTCOMES FOR STUDENTS WITH DISABILITIES?

One major feature of PL 105-17 is its least restrictive environment (LRE) provision to ensure that students receive the most inclusive placement feasible. However, current data indicate that segregated education for students with severe disabilities is common and, furthermore, is vastly inconsistent among states. The Sixteenth Annual Report to Congress on IDEA reported that 88% of the students with mental retardation in Vermont and in American Samoa attended general education classes (U.S. Department of Education, 1994a). The report also noted the other extreme with states like California at 3%, Minnesota at 4%, Pennsylvania at 2%, and New York at .5%. Such unevenness between geographic areas presents an untenable situation for students, their families, and the profession at large (Danielson & Bellamy, 1989). Because one must presume that children do not vary significantly based on place of residence, the data suggest that individualized education program (IEP) placement decisions are being influenced by factors other than the needs of each child. Clearly, a significant discrepancy exists among what the federal government envisioned, what some programs have achieved, and what is typically available to children with disabilities and their families at the state and local level.

Current implementation of the LRE provision continues to result in large numbers of children with identified special education and related services needs being placed in environments out of the general education classroom. The movement toward inclusive education is the most controversial interpretation of the LRE provision and the least utilized placement strategy. Inclusive education has been described by the National Association of State Boards of Education (NASBE) Special Education Study Group:

> At its core, inclusion means that students attend their home school along with their age and grade peers. A truly inclusive schooling environment is one in which students with the full range of abilities and disabilities receive their in-school educational services in the general education classroom with appropriate in-class support. In an inclusive education system, the proportion of students labeled for special services is relatively uniform for the schools within a particular school district and reflects the proportion of people with disabilities in society at large. In short, inclusion is not a place or a method of delivering instruction; it is a philosophy of supporting children in their learning that undergirds the entire system. It is part of the very culture of a school or school district and defines how students, teachers, administrators, and others view the potential of children. The inclusive philosophy of supported education espoused is truly grounded in the belief that all children can learn and achieve. (1995, p. 4)

Are schools complying with the law and attempting to ensure that students receive the services to which they are entitled? Judy Heumann, former Assistant Secretary of Education at the Office of Special Education and Rehabilitation Services (OSERS), commented on this:

> Although Part B of the IDEA has been in effect since 1975, nearly two thirds of the state plans submitted were not in compliance with the least restrictive environment requirements of the Act. Specifically, approximately two thirds of the plans when first submitted failed to include an adequate description of how the State Education Agency makes arrangements with public and private institutions to ensure that the least restrictive environment (LRE) requirements required by Part B are effectively implemented. Further, half of the plans originally submitted in 1991 did not ensure that public agencies only remove children with disabilities from the general educational environment when the nature or severity of the disability was such that education in regular classes with the use of supplementary aids and services could not be achieved satisfactorily. (1993, Amicus brief filed by OSERS in *Sacramento City Unified School District v. Holland*)

It is not surprising that much of the critique of segregated placement evolved in reference to students with the most severe disabilities. After all, this group of students has the distinction of being the least likely to be included in their district of residence, let alone in their school of residence and in a classroom with peers without disabilities. These were the same children who were most obviously excluded from education decades ago and were the plaintiffs in the court cases (e.g., *Pennsylvania Association for Retarded Children v. Commonwealth of Pennsylvania*, 1971) that eventually led to a national recognition of education as an inalienable right and the passage of PL 94-142.

The proliferation of segregated placements persists despite the range of information available to state and local programs on how to develop inclusive education programs (e.g., Fisher, Sax, & Pumpian, 1999; NASBE, 1992). Considerable support for the development of inclusive programs has emerged in recent years.

Literature describes philosophical bases as well as administrative and pedagogical strategies that can be used to move schools toward more inclusive practices (e.g., Halvorsen & Neary, 2001; Villa & Thousand, 2000). In addition, research efforts have produced literature on intervention practices that offer guidance for achieving positive outcomes within inclusive schools (e.g., McGregor & Vogelsberg, 1999).

Given this, what secondary school and postsecondary opportunities should be available for students with disabilities? The next section of this chapter provides an overview of the service delivery system design that is supported by current research and wise practices.

SERVICE DELIVERY QUESTIONS

Questions about service delivery should be considered for secondary school years (e.g., for students ages 14–18) and for postsecondary years (e.g., for students older than 18) as the options vary in each environment.

For the Secondary School Years

Before students with disabilities had access to the core curriculum in middle school and high school, community-based instruction (CBI) was a reasonable educational alternative. Given that students with significant disabilities could not easily gain access to the general education classroom, CBI provided the IEP team with a way to address functional skills. Today, in many schools and districts, students with and without disabilities have access to a rich and diverse curriculum with appropriate accommodations and modifications, as well as personal and technological supports (e.g., Jorgensen, 1998; Kennedy & Fisher, 2001). Since 1980, parents and professionals have learned a great deal about infusing functional skills into natural environments and age-appropriate activities (Giangreco, Cloninger, & Iverson, 1998). For example, science classes may not only reinforce basic math skills but also are ideal for teaching measurement, problem solving, and teamwork (i.e., functional skills).

One rationale for the emphasis on inclusive education at the secondary school level includes a knowledge base that students obtain in high school to prepare for their careers and adult life. High schools can provide a wealth of opportunities for the development of interpersonal relationships and effective work habits. By participating in the full range of activities offered as part of the curriculum and also extracurricular, they are better prepared with skills, experience, and relationships that lead to an integrated adult life (e.g., Falvey, 1995; Fisher, Sax, & Pumpian, 1998; Fisher et al. 1999; Schnorr, 1997). For example, district-level content and performance standards typically require that all students explore career options, participate in interviews and résumé writing, arrive to class on time, complete tasks assigned by a supervisor (teacher), use technology as a tool for learning, and learn to resolve conflict with peers. Obviously, students with disabilities benefit from these expectations as well. There is evidence that people with disabilities are more often dismissed from a job due to poor attendance and lack of social skills than because of their work skills (e.g., Shafer, Banks, & Kregel, 1991).

Furthermore, in general high school classes, students with disabilities can also gain membership (Schnorr, 1997), develop social relationships (Kennedy & Itkonen, 1994), encounter interesting core curriculum (Jorgensen, 1998), and increase their literacy skills (Ryndak, Morrison, & Sommerstein, 1999). Students without disabilities also benefit socially and academically from inclusive education (e.g., Staub & Peck, 1995). Beyond the immediate benefit of inclusive education for students without disabilities, those who are included in general schools will have more advantages later in life. As the current school-age population becomes the next generation of neighbors, friends, co-workers, employers, and parents of individuals with disabilities, inclusive education will not be questioned but rather will be used as a baseline for examining quality of life issues. Removing students with disabilities from high school classes today affects not only their postsecondary potential but also the circle of support available for years to come. We will never forget the high school junior who advocated for a peer with a disability in his English class to be hired for a part-time job, nor will we forget the high school senior who planned to become a pediatrician and who said to us, "I will never tell parents to institutionalize their children with disabilities."

For the Postsecondary School Years

Before natural supports were widely available in colleges or the workplace, students with disabilities rarely obtained postsecondary education or integrated employment (Mank, Buckley, Dean, & Cioffi, 1996). Today, competitive employment, supported living, and lifelong learning are expectations for adults with significant disabilities (Nisbet, 1992). School systems are responding to this need by establishing postsecondary (or transition) programs in the community (Johnson & Rusch, 1993; Martin, Mithaug, Oliphant, Husch, & Frazier, 2002). These programs provide the link from high school to a valued adult life for students with disabilities from ages 19–22. Many of these programs are located in the community to facilitate job development, job training, and continuing education, which cannot easily occur on the high school campus. Further, students use public transportation to go to work, college, or community events; increase their access to stores and public services; and adjust to schedules that mirror adult life.

For most people, postsecondary education and subsequent career development differs from their high school experience. Most people physically leave the high school campus, remain with their same-age peers, and pursue unique and challenging futures. Unfortunately, for many students with disabilities, there is little or no difference between high school and postsecondary education and career development. Students older than 18 years often remain on the high school campus, lose access to their peers without disabilities, and continue working on similar educational goals and objectives until they turn 21. Thus, consistent with the expectations for students without disabilities, a distinction must be made between high school (students 14–18 years of age) and postsecondary education (individuals older than 18).

Where people with disabilities spend time, with whom they interact, and what activities they choose are key considerations for program development and service delivery options. These choices must reflect the range of experiences that students began exploring in high school and expand to include career, continuing education, and social opportunities alongside their peers without disabilities. As students with disabilities increase the quality and quantity of their participation in these experiences during high school, the more likely they are to have access to the support required for success in postsecondary environments.

WHY ASSESS STUDENTS WITH SIGNIFICANT DISABILITIES?

How does information on the service delivery system, inclusive secondary schools, or postsecondary option fit into a book on assessment? Why would assessments matter to students with significant disabilities who are leaving the school system? This book provides a host of answers to these questions and more; however, it's important to consider some basics about assessment systems.

First, it is important to understand that students can be assessed for a wide variety of purposes, including

- Identifying individual student needs
- Improving instruction and program planning
- Evaluating service delivery programs
- Providing accountability information

The key is to know which type of assessment will give the information needed to help someone make a decision (e.g., the types of supports necessary in the workplace, the number of hours of independent living). Matching assessments to desired outcome information is critical, especially when negotiating systems change as Certo and colleagues point out in Chapter 9.

Second, it is important to understand that assessments are blunt tools. They are not sharp, precision instruments with which people operate. Using several types of assessments in concert with a conversation with the individual with a disability and his or her family and friends is critical. In other words, every assessment has its flaws. Beginning with a person-centered focus, using several approaches, and cross-referencing the results will reduce the chance that decisions are made *for* an individual rather than *with* that person. Sax (Chapter 2) and Craddock and Scherer (Chapter 7) focus on these issues—involve people, match appropriately, and cross-reference.

Third, the world of assessment is filled with "easy-to-use" tools that may not be consistent with the core values of the individual who is being assessed, his or her family and friends, the teachers or service coordinator, or other professionals. As Buswell and Sax (Chapter 4) and Wehmeyer (Chapter 3) point out, we know a lot about involving people with significant disabilities in their own transition assessments and planning. Although they acknowledge that it is not always easy, they make it clear that it is the right thing to do.

Fourth, you are legally required to assess students and develop transition plans. Why not make the plans meaningful and point students in the direction of a valued adult life? In other words, if time and money are going to be spent on assessments and planning, let's get it right. Assessments used should help and not hinder a person's chance of having places to live, work, and socialize that are valued. These assessments should identify the supports that are necessary for successful inclusion in community life rather than being used as evidence that a person is "too disabled" or needs "too much support" to be successful. Hughes and Carter (Chapter 5), Thoma and Held (Chapter 6), and Rogan, Grossi, and Gajewski (Chapter 8) provide a host of options for informal and alternative assessments that do exactly this—provide useful information leading to valued outcomes.

Fifth, and related to all four of the issues raised previously, the people who conduct these assessments must examine their own values. Everyone holds views of the world and of others. Some of these views must be questioned when planning with individuals with disabilities. Most commonly, people must examine their beliefs about community inclusion: Do I really believe that every person with a disability is entitled to a quality life that involves regular and sustained interactions with people without disabilities and who are also not paid to be there? Do I really believe that supports must be transparent and should be generic and natural whenever possible? Reflecting on these questions, Sax and Thoma (Chapter 10) share a story of a family who benefited from wise transition practices, and Danforth (Coda) provides a fable to consider while looking at the bigger picture of disability services and research.

People must also examine their beliefs about the multicultural and diverse world in which they live. If they hold negative or oppressive views based on gender, ethnicity, language, culture, religious beliefs, sexual orientation, or age, they must not allow these to cloud their decisions and practices. Taking the higher ground and believing in people and their rights to pursue their dreams is more important. Keeping these beliefs in check while assessing and planning for successful transitions is perhaps the most difficult thing to do. For more information about cross-cultural competence, see Lynch and Hanson (1998). You may want to engage in the activities they suggest prior to implementing the assessment strategies suggested in this book. All of the tools and wise practices in this book are based on an assumption that service delivery professionals are sensitive to the wishes, dreams, and hopes of people with disabilities and that they do not actively work against these dreams.

USING THIS BOOK

The authors have organized their chapters to best facilitate your adoption of wise practices in transition assessment. Each chapter begins with a story that illustrates issues faced by students and families as they approach the move from K–12 education to adult life. As you read the rest of this book, you should be asking yourself a series of questions. Some overarching questions that you may want to consider include

- How do we support individuals to identify outcomes that are important for their future?

- What information do we need in order to develop a plan with this student?
- How and from whom do we gather information?
- How do we decide what needs to happen in order to move from this starting point to a desired outcome?
- How do we translate this information into a seamless, effective plan?
- How do my own values and experiences affect the ways that I listen and apply this information?

Come "sit with us" as we explore the range of wise assessment practices that are used with people with significant disabilities who want to have great lives!

REFERENCES

Aune, E. (1991). A transition model for post-secondary bound students with learning disabilities. *Learning Disabilities Research and Practice, 6,* 177–187.

Braddock, D., & Mitchell, D. (1992). *Residential services and developmental disabilities in the United States.* Washington, DC: American Association on Mental Retardation.

Brown, F. (1991). Creative daily scheduling: A nonintrusive approach to challenging behaviors in community residences. *Journal of The Association for Persons with Severe Handicaps, 16,* 75–84.

Calculator, S.J., & Jorgensen, C.M. (1994). *Including students with severe disabilities in schools.* San Diego: Singular Publishing Group.

Cole, D.A., & Meyer, L.H. (1991). Social integration and severe disabilities: A longitudinal analysis of child outcomes. *Journal of Special Education, 25,* 340–351.

Danielson, L.C., & Bellamy, G.T. (1989). State variation in the placement of children with handicaps in segregated environments. *Exceptional Children, 55,* 448–455.

Education for All Handicapped Children Act of 1975, PL 94-142, 20 U.S.C. §§ 1400 et seq.

Evans, I.M., & Scotti, J.R. (1989). Defining meaningful outcomes for persons with profound disabilities. In F. Brown & D.H. Lehr (Eds.), *Persons with profound disabilities: Issues and practices* (pp. 83–107). Baltimore: Paul H. Brookes Publishing Co.

Falvey, M.A. (1995). *Inclusive and heterogeneous schooling: Assessment, curriculum, and instruction.* Baltimore: Paul H. Brookes Publishing Co.

Feinberg, W., & Soltis, J.F. (1992). *School and society.* New York: Teachers College Press.

Fisher, D., Sax, C., & Pumpian, I. (1998). Parent and careproviders' impressions of different educational models. *Remedial and Special Education, 19,* 173–180.

Fisher, D., Sax, C., & Pumpian, I. (1999). *Inclusive high schools: Learning from contemporary classrooms.* Baltimore: Paul H. Brookes Publishing Co.

Giangreco, M.F., Cloninger, C.J., & Iverson, V.S. (1998). *Choosing outcomes and accommodations for children: A guide to educational planning for students with disabilities* (2nd ed.). Baltimore: Paul H. Brookes Publishing Co.

Gilhool, T.K. (1976). Education: An inalienable right. In F. Weintraub, A. Abeson, J. Ballard, & M. Lavor (Eds.), *Public policy and the education of exceptional children* (pp. 14–21). Washington, DC: Council for Exceptional Children.

Halvorsen, A.T., & Neary, T. (2001). *Building inclusive schools: Tools and strategies for success.* Needham Heights, MA: Allyn & Bacon.

Heumann, J. (1993, November). *Comments on the Oberti teleconference.* Washington, DC: U.S. Department of Education, Office of Special Education and Rehabilitation Services.

Individuals with Disabilities Education Act (IDEA) Amendments of 1997, PL 105-17, 20 U.S.C. § 1400 et seq.

Johnson, J.R., & Rusch, F.R. (1993). Secondary special education and transition services: Identification and recommendations for future research and demonstration. *Career Development for Exceptional Individuals, 16,* 1–18.

Jorgensen, C.M. (1998). *Restructuring high schools for all students: Taking inclusion to the next level.* Baltimore: Paul H. Brookes Publishing Co.

Justen, J. (1976). Who are the severely handicapped?: A problem of definition. *AAESPH Review, 1,* 1–11.

Kennedy, C.H., & Fisher, D. (2001). *Inclusive middle schools.* Baltimore: Paul H. Brookes Publishing Co.

Kennedy, C.H., & Itkonen, T. (1994). Some effects of regular class participation on the social contacts and social networks of high school students with severe disabilities. *Journal of The Association for Persons with Severe Handicaps, 19,* 1–10.

Lynch, E.W., & Hanson, M.J. (Eds.). (1998). *Developing cross-cultural competence: A guide for working with children and their families* (2nd ed.). Baltimore: Paul H. Brookes Publishing Co.

Malakpa, S.W. (1994). Job placement of blind and visually impaired people with additional disabilities. *Re:view, 26,* 69–77.

Mank, D., Buckley, J., Dean, J., & Cioffi, A. (1996). Do social systems really change?: Retrospective interviews with state-supported employment systems-change projectors. *Focus on Autism and Other Developmental Disabilities, 11,* 243–250.

Martin, J., Mithaug, D., Oliphant, J., Husch, J., & Frazier, E.S. (2002). *Self-directed employment: A handbook for transition teachers and employment specialists.* Baltimore: Paul H. Brookes Publishing Co.

McDonnell, J.J., Hardman, M.L., McDonnell, A.P., & Kiefer-O'Donnell, R. (1995). *An introduction to persons with severe disabilities.* Needham Heights, MA: Allyn & Bacon.

McGregor, G., & Vogelsberg, R.T. (1999). *Inclusive schooling practices: Pedagogical and research foundations. A synthesis of the literature that informs best practices about inclusive schooling.* Baltimore: Paul H. Brookes Publishing Co.

Meyer, L.H., Peck, C.A., & Brown, L. (Eds.). (1991). *Critical issues in the lives of people with severe disabilities.* Baltimore: Paul H. Brookes Publishing Co.

Mithaug, D., Moriuchi, C., & Fanning, P. (1985). A report on the Colorado state-wide follow-up survey of special education students. *Exceptional Children, 51,* 397–404.

National Association of State Boards of Education (NASBE). (1992). *Winners all: A call for inclusive schools.* Report of the NASBE Study Group on Special Education. Washington, DC: Author.

National Association of State Boards of Education (NASBE). (1995). *Winning ways: Creating inclusive schools, classrooms, and communities.* Report of the NASBE Study Group on Special Education. Washington, DC: Author.

Nisbet, J. (Ed.). (1992). *Natural supports in school, at work, and in the community for people with severe disabilities.* Baltimore: Paul H. Brookes Publishing Co.

Oakes, J., & Lipton, M. (1990). *Making the best of schools: A handbook for parents, teachers, and policymakers.* New Haven: Yale University Press.

Pennsylvania Association for Retarded Citizens v. Commonwealth of Pennsylvania, 334 F. Supp. 1257. (E.D. Pa. 1971)

Ryndak, D.L., Morrison, A.P., & Sommerstein, L. (1999). Literacy before and after inclusion in general education settings: A case study. *Journal of The Association for Persons with Severe Handicaps, 24,* 5–22.

Schnorr, R.F. (1997). From enrollment to membership: "Belonging" in middle in high school classes. *Journal of The Association for Persons with Severe Handicaps, 22,* 1–15.

Shafer, M.S., Banks, P.D., & Kregel, J. (1991). Employment retention and career movement among individuals with mental retardation working in supported employment. *Mental Retardation, 29,* 103–110.

Stainback, S., Stainback, W., & Forest, M. (1989). *Educating all students in the mainstream of regular education.* Baltimore: Paul H. Brookes Publishing Co.

Staub, D., & Peck, C.A. (1995). What are the outcomes for nondisabled students? *Educational Leadership, 52*(4), 36–40.

U.S. Department of Education. (1993). *Fifteenth annual report to Congress on the implementation on the Individuals with Disabilities Education Act.* Washington, DC: Office of Special Education Programs.

U.S. Department of Education. (1994a). *Sixteenth annual report to Congress on the implementation on the Individuals with Disabilities Education Act.* Washington, DC: Office of Special Education Programs.

U.S. Department of Education. (1994b). *Strong families, strong schools: Building community partnerships for learning.* Washington, DC: Author.

Villa, R.A., & Thousand, J.S. (Eds.). (2000). *Restructuring for caring and effective education: Piecing the puzzle together* (2nd ed.). Baltimore: Paul H. Brookes Publishing Co.

Wagner, M. (1993). *The transition experiences of young people with disabilities: A summary of findings from the National Longitudinal Transition Study of Special Education Students.* Menlo Park, CA: SRI. (ERIC Document Reproduction Service No. EC 302 815)

Wehlage, G.G., & Rutter, R.A. (1986). Dropping out: How much do the schools contribute to the problem? *Teachers College Record, 87*(3), 364–392.

Wilson, K.G., & Daviss, B. (1994). *Redesigning education.* New York: Holt, Rinehart, & Winston.

Zigmond, N., & Thorton, H.S. (1985). Follow-up of post secondary age learning disabled graduates and dropouts. *Learning Disabilities Research, 1,* 50–55.

Person-Centered Planning

More than a Strategy

Caren L. Sax

METAPHORS FOR THE FUTURE

Shalamon, Bruce, and Ricardo were asked in a creative writing course to produce metaphors as they considered their futures beyond high school. They were all active in sports, so they thought immediately of things they used in the gym, including weights, treadmills, and exercise bicycles. Shalamon began by drawing a large barbell that held a number of weights on each side. He labeled the weights on each side, creating a balance of positive and not-so-positive traits, habits, and skills. He also added a stack of weights that included goals he wanted to pursue, such as finding an apprenticeship at a local high-technology firm, enrolling in community college, and traveling to a site where he could camp and river raft. Creating the images on paper made it easier for him to write his essay and to think about the characteristics that were needed to balance or support the pursuit of each goal.

Ricardo and Bruce talked about the contrast of using the treadmill and stationary bicycle with running on the beach and riding a bike on dirt trails. Because Bruce has difficulty thinking abstractly, they went to the gym to look at the equipment and figure out which pieces seemed to represent who they were and where they were going. They described the difference between "moving without getting anywhere" and "getting from Point A to Point B." They each saw themselves as people of action and expected that when they identified reachable goals, they would do what it took to meet and maybe exceed those goals. Working together on the project made it easier to articulate the details for the paper and portray themselves in a positive light.

PLANNING FOR THE FUTURE

People picture their lives and their futures using a variety of metaphors, symbols, and thought processes. In planning for their futures, these young men used familiar items to help them express their dreams and also their fears. Using metaphors was not only a valuable language lesson but also an introduction to taking charge of their lives for the future. Few people formulate clear pictures of who they are, who they want to be, where they want to go, and who they want to have for company without the contribution of others. Most young adults struggle with the balance of making decisions, taking responsibility for those decisions, and learning to exert more control over their lives. Person-centered planning is a vehicle toward this end.

Person-centered planning, personal futures planning, lifestyle planning, Making Action Plans (MAPS), and Planning Alternative Tomorrows with Hope (PATH), along with accompanying strategies, were created with the expectation that they would be implemented according to the philosophy and values on which they were based. Each approach actualizes the "vision of a just world, rich with diversity, in which every person's gifts are acknowledged, supported, valued; a world in which everyone is included, belongs, and makes valued contributions" (Pearpoint, O'Brien, & Forest, 1993, p. 1). More specifically, to remain true to the spirit by which these processes were designed, no one has a right to plan for another person's life without that individual's participation, permission, or request. This chapter provides a fresh look at individualizing person-centered planning strategies and provides examples of integrating the information into individualized education programs (IEPs), individualized transition plans (ITPs), individualized service plans (ISPs), individualized plans for employment (IPEs), and other planning documents. More important, it offers guidelines for using the information to help improve the quality of a person's real life (versus their life on paper).

PERSON-CENTERED VERSUS AGENCY-DRIVEN PLANNING

Much has been written about person-centered planning since the late 1980s (Allen & Shea, 1992; Forest & Lusthaus, 1989; Mount & Zwernik, 1988; O'Brien, 1987; Smull & Harrison, 1991; Vandercook, York, & Forest, 1989). The approach was originally "developed as a vehicle for including individuals with mental retardation more centrally in the process of developing goals and plans and to involve family members and other unpaid support people as partners with professionals" (Hagner, Helm, & Butterworth, 1996, p. 159). The hope was to maximize the level of community inclusion for individuals with mental retardation by fundamentally changing traditional agency-directed services. As the concept was applied to a broader population of individuals with disabilities, an increasing number of professionals were introduced to this planning methodology; however, it is still viewed too often as a *program* rather than as a philosophy-based *approach*. I hear from teachers and service providers who "use person-centered planning all the time" only to find out that, although the right questions may have been asked and the boxes may have been checked off, the services provided remain status quo. The range of services still tends to be limited by the funding and policy parameters, and the degree to which the services are truly individualized remains minimal.

In studies related to transition planning, person-centered approaches are particularly important to ensure the involvement of family and friends and other natural sources of support (Gallivan-Fenlon, 1994; Lichtenstein & Michaelides, 1993). Hagner and colleagues (1996), in their qualitative study of person-centered planning, followed six young adults with mental retardation in transition from school to adult life for 6 months beginning with the initial planning meeting. Despite the intent to conduct person-centered planning, those who organized and conducted the planning meetings did not always facilitate the ability of the focus individuals to drive the process. For example, the "individual's own views were sometimes ignored or reinterpreted, and the pace and tone of the meeting were sometimes dictated by others" (Hagner et al., 1996, p. 168). Inequalities in participation were also evident; that is, professionals often contributed more than the community participants. In addition, even though facilitators stated that comments should be made in a positive manner, they did not necessarily enforce this practice, leaving a negative impression of some of the meetings. Nevertheless, a number of unexpected positive outcomes seemed to result from the meetings, including the development of new relationships, more social activities, and job opportunities.

Person-centered planning requires equal participation, positive and clear communication, and active involvement of the focus individual. Clearly, the commitment must be to a long-term process rather than a single meeting, as direct and indirect outcomes are much more likely as a result of multiple meetings that take place over time and that build on the dynamic nature of the group. Furthermore, facilitators and participants must be willing to listen to the focus individual and be prepared to hear things that may not always match their preconceived ideas.

THE POWER OF PERSON-CENTERED PLANNING

Person-centered planning can be a powerful process when the issues mentioned previously are recognized and respected. I still remember when, as a relatively new teacher, I attended a school district seminar about building circles of friends around students with disabilities and then enlisting these new friends to help plan for the future. The practice of inclusive education was still new at that time, and the idea of helping students with significant disabilities identify and connect with their peers without disabilities presented different and awesome challenges. The examples of futures planning meetings that were provided in the seminar all sounded too scripted and idealistic and the quotes from young people engaged in the process sounded too good to be real. I was sure that the stories were greatly embellished. Several years later, when conducting my first person-centered planning meeting, I discovered that the stories were true.

The following descriptions of person-centered futures planning meetings illustrate ways to discover valuable assessment information about students facing transition. Each story has common threads that are essential components for creating positive action plans. These themes will be revisited throughout the book, as they are keys for a quality adult life.

Joanne Blazes the Trail

Joanne and her family were considered trailblazers in their community. As a young child in the 1970s, Joanne accompanied her sisters as they met and educated the neighbors about Down syndrome. Joanne was enrolled in the first preschool program offered for children with disabilities in the school district. She attended elementary and middle schools in the neighborhood, where she met students with and without disabilities even though she was based in a special education classroom. By the time she entered high school, times had changed, and she attended general education classes, making friends with many students on campus. Joanne's parents were very active in the school district as well as in the local center that provided services for individuals with developmental disabilities. Joanne was interested in a variety of activities, including dating and going to baseball games, movies, restaurants, and dances. She also had some definite ideas about her future.

I met Joanne and her family the year before Joanne was to graduate from high school. Her mother served as the school district parent liaison to inform families about services that were available to students who were transitioning into adult life. After getting to know Joanne and her family, I decided to help them organize a MAPS meeting to identify supports and resources that could enable Joanne to realize her dreams for the future.

Joanne made up the guest list with some advice from her parents. They hosted the meeting at their home, inviting friends, family, and assorted professionals to join in one of their traditional potluck dinners. This environment set the tone of the evening, raising the comfort level of all the participants but particularly for Joanne who was clearly pleased in her role as hostess. Joanne was typically quiet and did not necessarily enjoy being the center of attention, so this environment suited her well. The walls were cleared to make room for the large sheets of butcher paper on which the notes from her meeting were recorded.

We used the standard format, recording Joanne's history, places and activities she enjoyed, choices made by Joanne and those made for her, things that were working (i.e., that were motivating and interesting) and things that were not (i.e., that were boring, frustrating, or upsetting), and her dreams. An action plan was designed to identify specific tasks to be done by people who attended the meeting, along with a timeline for both short-term and long-term goals. Most of the information gathered that night went directly into Joanne's IEP, providing clear direction for her activities.

A series of potluck meetings were held during the next few years as Joanne exited the school district, enrolled in community college courses, worked at several jobs, and dated at least two different men. She eventually moved into an apartment with her sister and her nephew where she began hosting her own potluck dinners to continue the family tradition. Joanne decided when she wanted to have people gather to help with major decisions. The guest list changed over the years and the process became increasingly informal. Joanne was truly living her dreams and taught friends and professionals alike a great deal about the power of person-centered planning. She learned to be more assertive in expressing her opinions and preferences. When she asked for advice, she listened to others but also followed her own heart and mind in making decisions.

The success of Joanne's meetings demonstrates the importance of context and choosing the appropriate participants in the process; that is, those who listen more than talk and who withhold judgment when necessary. Joanne's story also illustrates the importance of planning over a number of years. With each new meeting, Joanne was able to exert more control over the guest list, focus for discussion, and tone of the meeting. She continued in the role of a trailblazer, demonstrating self-determination before ever hearing the term.

Stephen Uploads His Future

After facilitating meetings for Joanne and a number of other people, I began to think about customizing meetings around a theme that might be more meaningful to the focus individual, particularly for those who had more difficulty with abstract thinking or traditional communication. When I was asked to facilitate a meeting for Stephen, who has autism, I knew I needed another approach.

Stephen was a junior in his neighborhood high school at the time of his first futures planning meeting. The purpose of the meeting was twofold: one, to help Stephen get better connected socially, and two, to begin designing activities and experiences that would lead him to his future goals of attending college and working in a job where he could use his computer skills. At the time, Stephen was not known for his ability to interact well with his peers. Other students were intrigued by his behavior, impressed by his computer skills, and often puzzled about how to talk to him. There were no clear beginnings or endings to his conversations. He often entered a room already talking and typically left without warning.

The standard MAPS format was not likely to interest him, so I created a series of computer screens on large sheets of paper to provide a familiar and favorite context. Thinking in the abstract was challenging for Stephen, so the language of the meeting and accompanying graphics were all computer related. The whole session was limited to four categories (see Figure 2.1). The first screen, *open file*, was used to get a sense of who Stephen was from his perspective as well as from those of the participants. The next screen was used to identify *info to save*, that is, things that were going well for him. Stephen was able to explain what worked for him, such as receiving an explanation behind a direction instead of simply being told not to do something. Some of his peers told Stephen that it was also his responsibility to ask for help instead of leaving the room or becoming frustrated. The conversation helped the students to understand that these skills were difficult for Stephen, that he needed to study and practice in order to improve these skills.

The third screen opened the conversation of *info to edit*. Stephen's teacher talked about Stephen's frustration in dealing with last-minute changes to his routine and his habit of ignoring directions when he did not want to listen. Some of the students talked about escape strategies that he might try, and how they, too, often felt frustrated in certain classes. Stephen added that he did not always need a peer tutor in a class to correct him; rather, sometimes he just needed a friend.

Bytes About Stephen

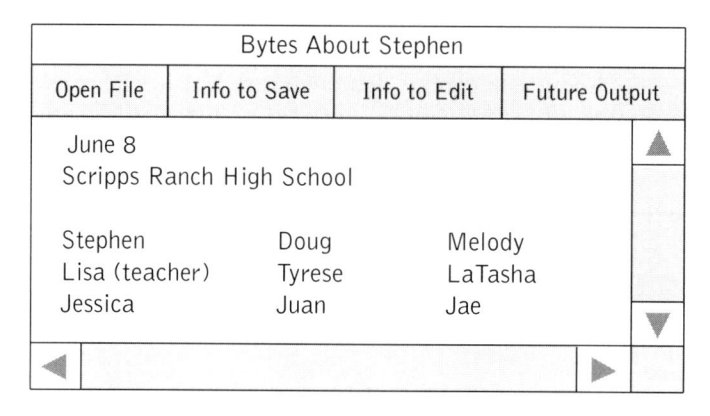

Open File	Info to Save	Info to Edit	Future Output

June 8
Scripps Ranch High School

Stephen	Doug	Melody
Lisa (teacher)	Tyrese	LaTasha
Jessica	Juan	Jae

Open File

Open File	Info to Save	Info to Edit	Future Output

Inquisitive	Personable
Intelligent	Analytical
Considerate	Unique
Caring	Imaginative
Outgoing	Outspoken
Highly motivated	Talented at horse riding

Info to Save

Open File	Info to Save	Info to Edit	Future Output

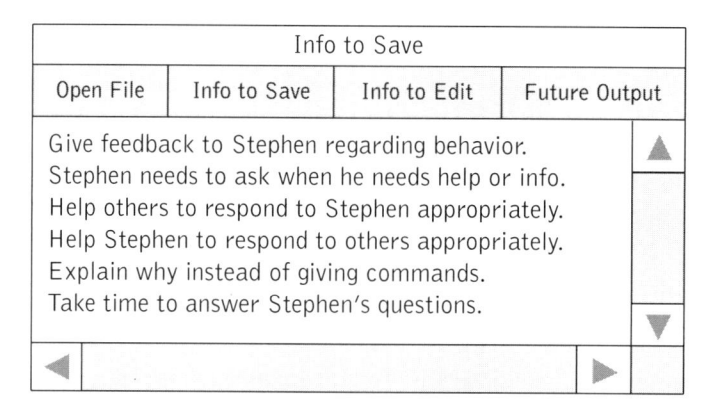

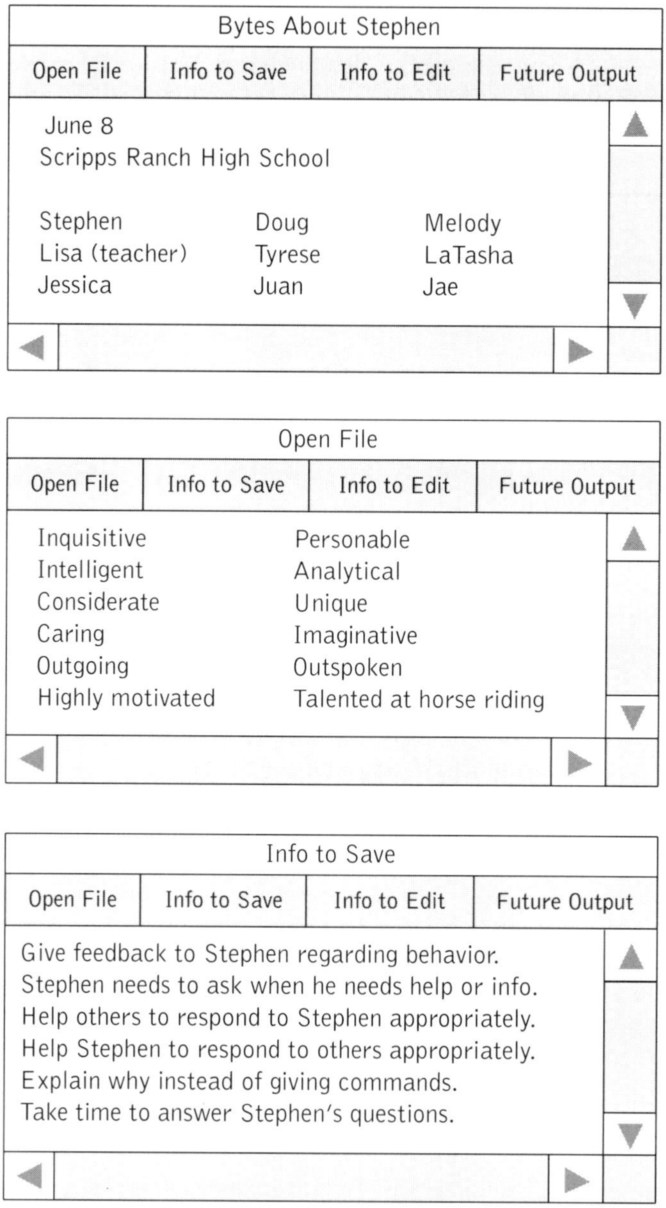

Give feedback to Stephen regarding behavior.
Stephen needs to ask when he needs help or info.
Help others to respond to Stephen appropriately.
Help Stephen to respond to others appropriately.
Explain why instead of giving commands.
Take time to answer Stephen's questions.

Figure 2.1. Customized futures planning with Stephen and high school peers.

The final screen was to record brainstorming on *future output*. Most of these goals were short term, to be accomplished during the summer. They included learning to drive, applying for a job, and having a pool party. Stephen seemed pleased with the outcomes and was invited to a number of social events as a result of the meeting.

Info to Edit			
Open File	Info to Save	Info to Edit	Future Output

Has trouble with taking "orders" on spur of the moment things
Blows things out of proportion
Does not need peer tutor; would rather have friend
Uses escape strategies
Uses ignoring

Future Output			
Open File	Info to Save	Info to Edit	Future Output

Attend summer school if necessary
Learn to drive
Swim and go to a pool party
Apply for a job at a computer company
Go to the movies
Call friends to go to the zoo and the beach

As in Joanne's case, ideas from this session were incorporated directly into Stephen's IEP goals. His peers offered useful advice to help Stephen communicate his frustrations more clearly, and the conversations helped them to see Stephen's skills as well as his needs. Their recommendations were much more likely to be used by Stephen than the generic-sounding objectives written year after year addressing his lack of social skills. Many events that followed the original meeting led to a successful transition for Stephen, who applied to a 4-year university to major in computer science. Several years later, he was hired as computer support staff for a university-based project. He earned his driver's license and began making plans to move into his own apartment.

The essential components that appeared in Stephen's planning experience initially led him to pursue social skills with the same intensity and precision that he approached learning computer skills. Specifically, the group encouraged him to express his frustrations and opinions and listened to his ideas on how things might be improved. He often perseverated on topics such as the value of homework and the unfairness of every teacher scheduling assignments and tests at the same time; however, his peers figured out ways of addressing his questions while leading him to other topics. Involvement in this and other follow-up meetings helped Stephen to understand the importance of self-advocacy and the pay-off when decisions are made with him instead of for him.

PERSON-CENTERED AND PERSONALIZED PLANNING

Other personalized themes included a futures planning meeting for a young man, Hector, who was enamored by Hollywood stars and movie trivia. He had a job at a movie theater taking tickets and directing people to the right screen. Hector wanted to move onto a local college campus so that he could take classes and have more social opportunities. His person-centered planning documents began with a theater marquee, featuring his name in lights (see Figure 2.2 on pages 22–23). The *cast of players* included friends, transition teachers and paraprofessionals, a co-worker, and representatives from adult service delivery agencies. Together the group described the *working scene,* the *living scene,* the school scene, and the *social scene.* Each scene was introduced with a director's board and listed the current status as *now showing* and the future goals as *coming attractions*. The action plan included supporting roles and behind-the-scenes resources.

This approach kept Hector focused and also sparked the rest of the group into designing their own meetings. The group members realized that almost everyone who is beginning college needs some help with mapping out his or her future, and they believed Hector's meeting was valuable. The meeting also helped them to understand the supports and resources that were available for Hector and why he needed access to them when necessary. Because Hector's disabilities were not as obvious, it was difficult for some of his peers to understand his inconsistent behavior. This meeting helped with their understanding yet did so in a respectful way that included Hector. Hector helped to run the meeting, providing him an avenue for developing his own skills in self-advocacy.

Person-centered planning was also used with Manuel, a young man with cerebral palsy. The floor plan of a local home improvement business was used to guide his futures planning meeting. Each aisle was labeled according to where he could find the tools to succeed in his goals and dreams. As this was one of his favorite places, Manuel was thrilled with the idea. Of course, I brought the actual tools to this meeting, so that each member of the group could choose a tool and identify a characteristic that represented Manuel's skills, dreams, or preferences. Friends and families discussed everything from his ability to shed light on new topics (flashlight) to trying to think about long-range goals (measuring tape). The meeting was interactive and very concrete in the way that plans were designed and language was used. Manuel, despite his own limited ability to communicate, was a full participant in the process.

The caution with any and all of these approaches is to resist the temptation to get caught up in the theme, enjoy the meeting, and then go back to business as usual. For example, I once conducted a person-centered planning meeting at the request of a family who was having some difficulties in understanding all the options available for their son. It was clear that they were feeling pressured to place their son, Jamal, in a segregated worksite, although that was not their first choice. The discussion included a wide range of future options after identifying Jamal's strengths, interests, and experiences, illustrated through the use of a PATH process. Short-term (1 week, 1 month, 3 months) and long-term (1 year, 5 years) goals were pictured, as were the steps and supports required to reach these goals. The drawings were colorful and entertaining, and the attendees found themselves thinking more creatively. The case manager seemed impressed with the process and joined in the very positive conversation, then shocked everyone by saying, "Okay, let's get back to talking about the place for Jamal that is available. When do you want him to start?"

Even the most creative processes are not enough without a definite plan of action that is person centered, not systems directed. The meeting is only one step. Person-centered planning is a way of thinking and provides a clear direction that is identified by the individual. Without the commitment of the participants to listen to the individual and respect his or her choices, the lives of people with disabilities are not likely to gain in quality.

VALUES-DRIVEN PLANNING

As Doug Fisher and I stated in Chapter 1, professionals must examine their own values, particularly as they are positioned to help individuals with disabilities determine their futures. Having professionals conduct their own futures planning session is a useful strategy to develop a better understanding of the process and can also help to reflect on values, biases, and assumptions that may affect the way in which they listen and understand. Participating in a person-centered planning process is not always easy, nor is it always comfortable, but it can result in a clear path toward a quality life. Thinking about change often creates anxiety; experiencing change when the resources and supports are not in place can create chaos.

Using a person-centered approach to assess students who are exiting the school system and entering the adult world should be a multipronged effort. Assessing the student is one facet; assessing the environment that they are entering is another. Matching people with desired friends, jobs, social activities, assistive technology, or other accommodations requires that teachers, families, and other services providers become much more savvy about identifying resources in the community that best match the needs and interests of the student. Creating opportunities while identifying supports and resources is a balancing act, one that takes into account the individual's personality, personal support network, and knowledge of rights as well as responsibilities.

CLOSING THOUGHTS

Assessing, or "sitting with," people as described previously, can provide continuity for the person-centered planning process. People change, their family situations change, and their hopes and dreams change. Planning takes place throughout an individual's life and the skills to participate in and direct this planning process improve over time. In order to make this approach meaningful and worthwhile, all parties must be committed to the philosophy and belief that individuals with significant disabilities deserve the opportunity to direct the path of their lives. Dreams cannot be fulfilled if they are neither conceptualized nor pursued; students, families, and professionals all have a responsibility to encourage those dreams.

NOW SHOWING

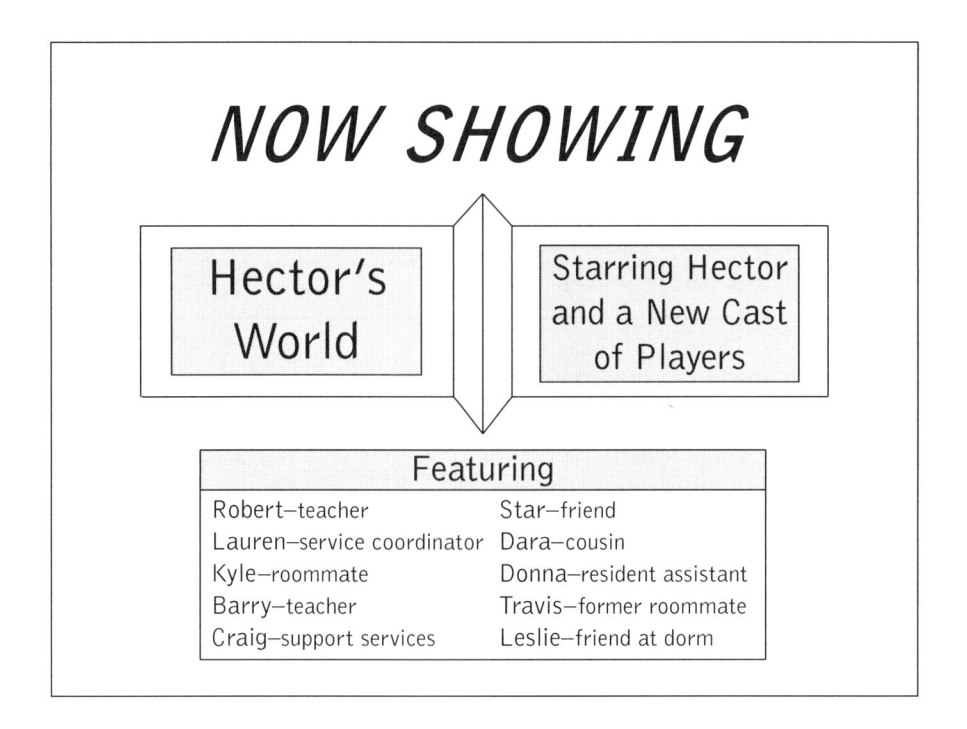

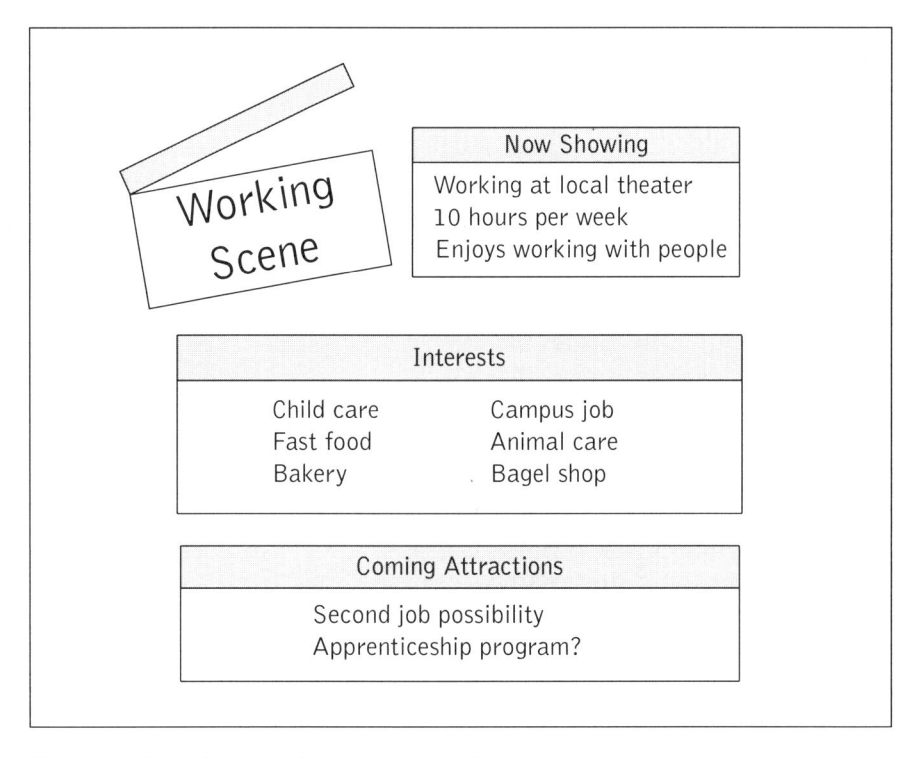

Hector's World

Starring Hector and a New Cast of Players

Featuring	
Robert—teacher	Star—friend
Lauren—service coordinator	Dara—cousin
Kyle—roommate	Donna—resident assistant
Barry—teacher	Travis—former roommate
Craig—support services	Leslie—friend at dorm

Working Scene

Now Showing
Working at local theater
10 hours per week
Enjoys working with people

Interests	
Child care	Campus job
Fast food	Animal care
Bakery	Bagel shop

Coming Attractions
Second job possibility
Apprenticeship program?

Figure 2.2. Hector's movie-style person-centered planning notes.

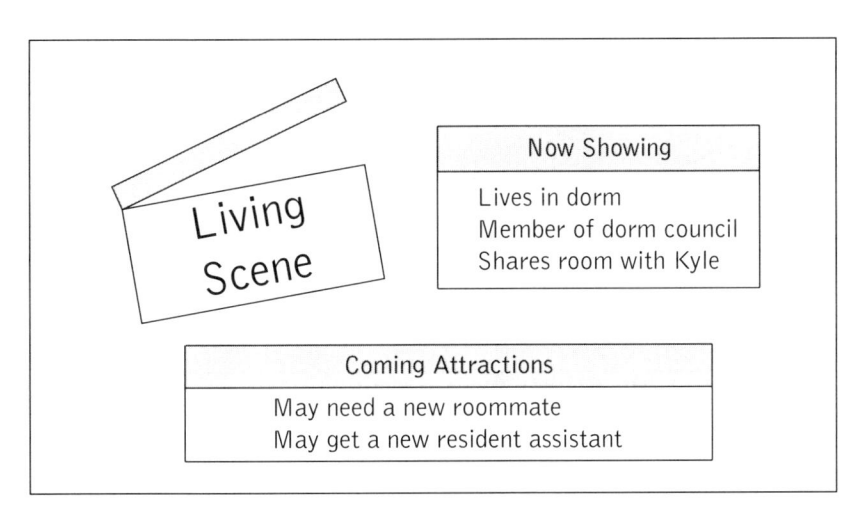

Living Scene

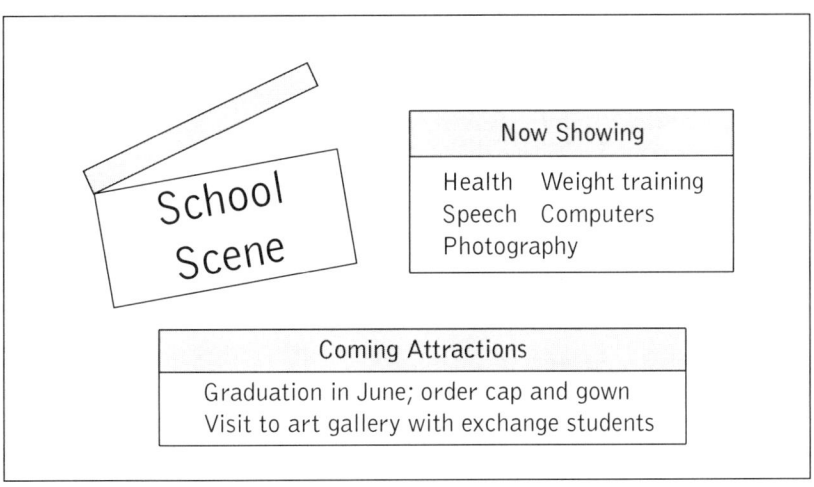

Now Showing
Lives in dorm
Member of dorm council
Shares room with Kyle

Coming Attractions
May need a new roommate
May get a new resident assistant

School Scene

Now Showing
Health   Weight training
Speech   Computers
Photography

Coming Attractions
Graduation in June; order cap and gown
Visit to art gallery with exchange students

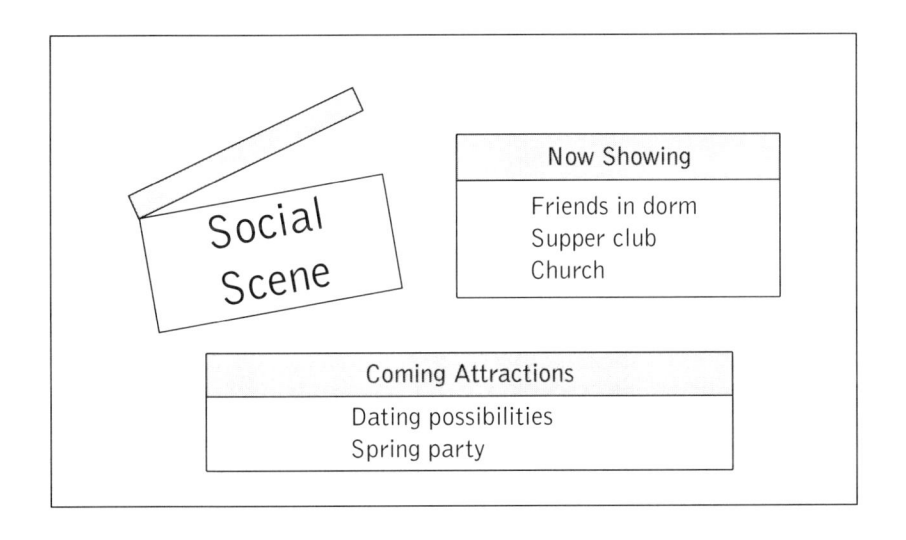

Social Scene

Now Showing
Friends in dorm
Supper club
Church

Coming Attractions
Dating possibilities
Spring party

REFERENCES

Allen, W.T., & Shea, J.R. (1992). *Explorations: Selected excerpts from a survey of quality-of-life measurements for the state of Colorado.* Napa, CA: Allen, Shea, and Associates.

Forest, M., & Lusthaus, E. (1989). Promoting educational equality for all students: Circles and maps. In S. Stainback, W. Stainback, & M. Forest (Eds.), *Educating all students in the mainstream of regular education* (pp. 43–58). Baltimore: Paul H. Brookes Publishing Co.

Gallivan-Fenlon, A. (1994). "Their senior year": Family and service provider perspectives on the transition from school to adult life for young adults with disabilities. *Journal of The Association for Persons with Severe Handicaps, 19,* 11–23.

Hagner, D., Helm, D.T., & Butterworth, J. (1996). "This is your meeting": A qualitative study of person-centered planning. *Mental Retardation, 34*(3), 159–171.

Lichtenstein, S., & Michaelides, N. (1993). Transition from school to young adulthood: Four case studies of young adults labeled mentally retarded. *Career Development for Exceptional Individuals, 16,* 183–195.

Mount, B., & Zwernik, K. (1988). *It's never too early, it's never too late: A booklet about personal futures planning.* Minnesota Governor's Planning Council on Developmental Disabilities (Pub. No. 421–88–109).

O'Brien, J. (1987). A guide to life-style planning: Using the activities catalog to integrate services and natural support systems. In B. Wilcox & G.T. Bellamy (Eds.), *A comprehensive guide to the activities catalog: An alternative curriculum for youth and adults with severe disabilities* (pp. 175–189). Baltimore: Paul H. Brookes Publishing Co.

Pearpoint, J., O'Brien, J., & Forest, M. (1993). *PATH: A workbook for planning positive possible futures.* Toronto, Ontario, Canada: Inclusion Press.

Smull, M., & Harrison, S. (1991). *Supporting people with severe reputations in the community: A handbook for trainers.* Baltimore: Johns Hopkins University, Department of Pediatrics.

Vandercook, T., York, J., & Forest, M. (1989). The McGill Action Planning System (MAPS): A strategy for building the vision. *Journal of The Association for Persons with Severe Handicaps, 14*(3), 205–215.

3

Self-Determined Assessment
Critical Components for Transition Planning

Michael L. Wehmeyer

CECILE TAKES CHARGE

Cecile approached her graduation from high school with some fear and trepidation, as might be expected, but also with a sense of purpose and control that was not evident in some of her peers. They had suddenly realized that school would be ending in just a few weeks, and they had no idea what they were going to do. Cecile, however, had been planning for this event for at least 5 years. She allowed herself to experience a brief sense of pride over that thought—the fact that she had been planning for her life and her future. Five years ago, when Ms. Crossland had informed her that she was going to receive something called transition services that would help her plan for her future, Cecile had a hard time thinking that far ahead (after all, the eighth-grade prom was right around the corner—who could think past that?) and, to be perfectly honest, she figured it was just another "school thing" that would be boring and useless. When Ms. Crossland suggested that she, Cecile, would want to become involved in the planning for her future, she was even more skeptical. When had adults really listened to her anyway?

But, this time it was different. Throughout her eighth-grade year, Cecile worked with Ms. Crossland to make sure that she had some skills and knowledge about how to plan for her future. This process started with learning about transition, what meetings are for, what types of planning would take place, and how and why to set transition goals. Her first transition planning meeting was something she would remember for a long time because she had several ideas for her individualized education program (IEP) that the team took and included in her goals and objectives. Then, Ms. Crossland asked her to think about what skills and knowledge she needed to learn to get where she wanted in life. Actually, it took a few years for her to really get to know what she wanted to do, where she wanted to live, what type of work she wanted to do, and all those things. She certainly didn't do it alone. By her transition meeting during her junior year in high school, there was a whole roomful of people she had invited, from the vocational counselor who was helping her get the job she was interested in, to her parents, to members of her synagogue.

Sure, there were a lot of evaluations and assessments to complete, but because she was in charge of gathering information about herself, it wasn't boring! She became better at setting goals and tracking them. She learned more about problem solving and decision making. She even used her new self-advocacy skills to run for student council vice president during her senior year. Her senior year had been great, and she hated to see it end. But she didn't really see it as an end. She saw it as a beginning, a beginning that was 5 years and lots of meetings and hard work in the making.

USE OF MULTIPLE APPROACHES

Cecile's story is an example of the promise of facilitating student self-determination in the transition assessment and planning process. Students need to be prepared to make decisions for their own lives, and the transition process is a great time for them to practice and fine-tune their skills. This chapter introduces strategies that students, teachers, and parents can use to help students make wise choices for their lives.

Clark (1996) suggested that it is important for transition assessment to include multiple approaches, including standardized tests, interviews, direct observation, and criterion-referenced assessment. Clark identified assessments that are available for transition planning and evaluation, including 1) learning style inventories, 2) academic achievement tests, 3) adaptive behavior scales, 4) aptitude tests, 5) interest inventories, 6) personality scales, 7) quality of life scales, 8) social skills inventories, 9) vocational/employability scales, 10) vocational skills assessments, and 11) transition knowledge and skills inventories. Although many of these instruments are not specific to transition, they can provide information on a range of student strengths, limitations, knowledge, skills, interests, and preferences and, thus, enable transition planners to create a comprehensive picture of the student.

Clark (1996) also listed the types of informal assessment from which transition-related decisions can be made, including 1) situational or observational learning styles assessments; 2) curriculum-based assessment; 3) observational reports from teachers, employers, and family members; 4) situational assessments in home, community, and work environments; 5) environmental assessments; 6) personal future planning activities; 7) structured interviews with students; 8) structured interviews with parents, guardians, advocates, or peers; 9) adaptive, behavior, or functional skill inventories; 10) social histories; 11) employability, independent living, and personal-social skills rating scales; and 12) technology or vocational education skills assessments.

Self-Determined Assessment

Again, these assessment procedures enable planners to form a complete picture of student needs, interests, and abilities by gathering input from multiple sources; however, in addition to using these traditional components of transition assessment, transition programs also need to include assessments that identify student strengths and limitations in self-determination skill areas and that incorporate student self-report measures and student self-evaluation procedures into the assessment process.

ASSESSING STUDENT INTERESTS AND PREFERENCES

The transition services process mandated by the Individuals with Disabilities Education Act (IDEA) Amendments of 1997 (PL 105-17) begin with students' needs, taking into account students' interests and preferences. As such, the logical first step in the transition assessment process is to identify student interests and preferences, a key feature in assessment in self-determination as well. The most straightforward means of assessing student preferences is to interview the student and his or her friends or family members. For students who cannot easily articulate their preferences, educational planners will need to go beyond interviews to provide more systematic means of assessing student preferences and interests. Hughes, Pitkin, and Lorden (1998) conducted a review of such strategies, summarized in the following sections.[1]

Activation of a Microswitch

Some students have limited verbal skills and very little use of their arms or legs. It is difficult for them to express preferences in conventional manners (e.g., verbally, picking up a preferred item, engaging in a chosen activity). One strategy for these students involves teaching them to use whatever physical movement they can make to activate a microswitch to indicate a choice among one or two items or activities.

Approach Toward an Object

Another strategy for assessing the preferences and choices of people with limited verbal skills is to observe whether they approach an object when it is presented. One or more objects or events can be presented at a time to a student. Assessing preferences using the approach strategy may easily be used with any student, with or without a disability. A teacher simply needs to note across time which items, activities, materials, or events students tend to approach in a situation in which all options are equally and readily available (e.g., free time).

---

[1]From Wehmeyer, M.L., Agran, M., & Hughes, C. (1998). *Teaching self-determination to students with disabilities: Basic skills for successful transition* (pp. 104–107). Baltimore: Paul H. Brookes Publishing Co.; adapted by permission.

Verbalizations, Gestures, and Affect

For students who have expressive communication skills, indications of preferences and choices may include a variety of expressive behavior, including verbalizations, manual signing, physical gestures, vocalizations, or physical affect.

Physical Selection of an Item

The preferences of students with disabilities also can be assessed by observing whether they physically select (e.g., pick up) an item when it is presented. This strategy requires that the item be present in the environment for the student to select, which may limit the variety of choices that can be offered; however, the range of options can be expanded by presenting items representational of an activity, event, or situation. For example, a ticket to a baseball game could represent the opportunity to see a game or a book of coupons could represent the opportunity to go grocery shopping.

Task Performance

Another strategy for measuring preference that requires the physical presence of a choice item is observing a student's performance of a specific task. Wacker, Berg, Wiggins, Muldoon, and Cavanaugh (1985) used task performance as a preference assessment strategy when they observed the performance of five students on instructional tasks (e.g., range of motion exercises). When the students performed a targeted behavior, they were given access to a potentially preferred item. Items were varied across performance sessions in order that the effect on performance of different items could be compared. Increases in task performance were associated with access to specific items for all students. Because of the reinforcing effect these items had on task performance, they were considered to be preferred.

Time Engaged with an Item

Preference for items or activities also has been inferred from the amount of time a student has continued to be engaged with one item in comparison to time spent with other items or activities. Kennedy and Haring (1993) used a time engagement strategy when they assessed the preferences of four students with multiple disabilities. Items such as a computer game or jigsaw puzzle were suggested by the students' teachers as likely either to be preferred or not by each student. The items were then placed one at a time on each student's wheelchair laptop, and the amount of time the student was engaged with the item during a 1-minute opportunity was noted and compared with time spent with other items. Findings showed that each student had preferences for interacting more with some items than others.

Observing Students' Responses Over Time

In assessing a student's preferences, it is important to observe the choices he or she makes over an extended period of time. The studies reviewed by Hughes and colleagues (1998) indicated that student preferences may vary across opportunities to choose. For example, a student may prefer to listen to rock music for several weeks in a row and then change to a preference for country music. Shifts in preference should not be surprising when one considers that, after recent access to one type of object or activity, a student may become bored or disinterested and wish for a change. In addition, although some students tend to pick the same options for a lengthy period of time before switching to another, some prefer to vary their choices frequently. Consequently, preferences may not be evident immediately. To get a true picture of a student's preferences, it is important to observe the choices a student makes over an extended period of time. A teacher then can estimate the percentage of times a particular option was chosen out of the total number of opportunities. Those options chosen a higher percentage of time than others likely are preferred by a student.

It is necessary to sample a student's interests and preferences often because such interests or preferences do change over time. Once student interests and preferences in transition areas are established, assessment should focus on identifying student skill areas and areas of instructional needs. Accomplishing this in relation to self-determination will involve a combination of assessment activities. As discussed subsequently, this needs to be accomplished within the context of an *empowerment evaluation* framework. Transition assessment then becomes a collaborative effort, combining the input of the student and other significant stakeholders.

ASSESSING INSTRUCTIONAL NEEDS IN SELF-DETERMINATION

It is important to note that the assessment of instructional needs in self-determination should embody key features that may not be a component of traditional transition assessment activities. That is, assessment in self-determination should be based within an empowerment evaluation framework, be future-oriented, employ multiple measurement techniques that include participant self-report indicators, and involve key stakeholders in the process.

Empowerment evaluation involves the "use of concepts, techniques and findings to foster improvement and self-determination" (Fetterman, 1996, p. 4). According to Fetterman, empowerment evaluation has "an unambiguous value orientation, designed to help people help themselves and improve their programs using a form of self-evaluation and reflection" (1996, p. 5). It is, by necessity, a collaborative group activity with a focal point on the individual as an evaluator as well as being evaluated, thus emphasizing self-evaluation and self-directed assessment. Similarly, assessment in self-determination needs to have the same unambiguous orientation toward enabling people to help themselves.

Like self-determination, quality of life is a multidimensional construct, and researchers and practitioners can turn to struggles to measure that construct to provide direction for pursuits in measuring self-determination. Specifically, as is the case in measuring quality of life, measurement in self-determination must involve multiple indicators that include participant observation, personal interviews, subjective and objective indicators, and standardized instruments. Only when there are rich sources of data generated from these multiple methods and perspectives can researchers and practitioners begin to adequately measure self-determination.

Determining instructional and curricular needs in the area of self-determination will involve a combination of standardized and informal procedures incorporating input from multiple sources, including the student, his or her family, professionals, and others. Informal procedures will be similar to those described previously by Clark (1996). There are a few standardized measures of self-determination and its component elements that could be used to identify instructional and curricular needs, some of which are tied to instructional curricula. For example, the self-determination curriculum Steps to Self-Determination: A Curriculum to Help Adolescents Learn to Achieve Their Goals (Field & Hoffman, 1996) provides criterion-referenced assessment instruments, including a student self-report measure.

Likewise, students involved in the Next S.T.E.P. (Student Transition and Educational Planning) curriculum (Halpern et al., 1997; described subsequently) complete the Transition Skills Inventory, a 72-item rating instrument assessing how well the student is doing in four transition areas: 1) personal life, 2) jobs, 3) education and training, and 4) living on one's own. The student's self-evaluation of these areas is combined with similar evaluations by his or her teacher and a family member to form a basis for future transition planning activities. Students are encouraged to discuss differences of opinion between the teacher or family member evaluations and their own self-evaluation and to resolve these discrepancies either before or during the transition planning meeting.

The ChoiceMaker materials, designed to promote student involvement in educational planning and decision making, include an assessment component that can be used to identify student self-determination needs. The ChoiceMaker Self-Determination Transition Assessment (Martin & Marshall, 1996) is tied to the ChoiceMaker curriculum and provides teachers an opportunity to rate student skills and student opportunities to perform such skills in areas like choosing goals and taking action.

Another instrument to assess student self-determination is The Arc's Self-Determination Scale (Wehmeyer & Kelchner, 1995). This scale is a 72-item self-report measure that provides data on each of the four essential characteristics of self-determination identified by Wehmeyer and colleagues as defining self-determined behaviors (Wehmeyer, Kelchner, & Richards, 1996). The scale measures 1) student autonomy, including the student's independence and the degree to which he or she acts on the basis of personal beliefs, values, interests, and abilities; 2) student self-regulation, including interpersonal cognitive problem solving and goal setting, and task performance; 3) psychological empowerment; and 4) student self-realization. The Arc's Self-Determination Scale was normed with 500 students with and without cognitive disabilities in rural, urban, and suburban school districts across five states. The scale has been used:

1. To conduct research on the relationship between self-determination and positive adult outcomes (Wehmeyer & Schwartz, 1997) as well as quality of life variables (Wehmeyer & Schwartz, 1998)
2. To examine the relationship between self-determination and environmental factors (Wehmeyer & Bolding, 1999, in press)
3. To validate instructional strategies to promote self-determination (Wehmeyer, Palmer, Agran, Mithaug, & Martin, 2000) and create materials to promote student-directed transition planning (Wehmeyer & Lawrence, 1995)

However, the primary purpose of the scale is to enable students with cognitive disabilities to self-assess strengths and limitations in the area of self-determination and to provide students and teachers with a tool they can use jointly to determine goals and instructional programming to promote self-determination.

Another measure of self-determination is the American Institute of Research Self-Determination Scale (Wolman, Campeau, DuBois, Mithaug, & Stolarski, 1994), which measures individual capacity for and opportunity to practice self-determination. There are educator, student, and parent forms of the scale, and the results of each can be used to develop a profile of a student's level of self-determination, identify areas of strength and areas needing improvement, identify educational goals and objectives, and develop strategies to build student capacity and increase students' opportunities to become self-determined.

All of the previously mentioned assessments measure global self-determination; however, there are also numerous instruments that measure individual essential characteristics or component elements of self-determined behavior. For example, the Autonomous Functioning Checklist (AFC; Sigafoos, Feinstein, Damond, & Reiss, 1988) is a parent-completed checklist designed to measure the behavioral autonomy of adolescents. The scale has 78 items and is subdivided into four subscales: self and family care, management, recreational activity, and social and vocational activity. Lewis and Taymans (1992) used the AFC to examine the autonomous functioning of adolescents with learning disabilities.

ENABLING STUDENTS TO SELF-DIRECT LEARNING AND ASSESSMENT

Returning to some of the unique features of assessment in self-determination, it would be insufficient to limit a discussion of transition assessment and self-determination to strategies and instruments that simply *assess* transition interests, preferences, and needs. Indeed, as emphasized earlier in the chapter, there is a critical need to actively involve the student in the transition assessment process. Most of the instruments discussed earlier are student report measures designed to provide a vehicle for students to self-assess needs related to self-determination and transition. There are several instructional programs that provide a structure by which students can be taught to take greater control over their educational experiences.

The emphasis on participatory planning and student involvement in planning and decision making is in response to, and in contrast with, the historical role of students in educational planning and decision making, a role that has been one of passivity and inactivity. The Education for All Handicapped Children Act of 1975 (PL 94-142) and all subsequent amendments provided for students' involvement in IEP decisions "whenever appropriate" and, as Gillespie and Turnbull (1983) have pointed out, this was too frequently interpreted to mean that student involvement was not appropriate or necessary. As a result, student involvement in educational planning and decision making became haphazard at best, and students were essentially outsiders to the educational decision-making process. Van Reusen and Bos (1990) concluded that "student involvement [in educational planning], even at the secondary level, is for the most part either nonexistent or passive" (p. 30). This is in spite of evidence that student involvement can have positive effects on student achievement, outcomes, and motivation and that for the most part, educators agree that students can benefit from greater involvement in transition planning. Walker and Shaw (1995) found that special educators perceived student involvement in transition planning to be low but felt such involvement to be desirable.

The 1997 amendments to IDEA, PL 105-17, did, however, include language indicating that students must be invited to and be a critical part of transition planning. As a result of this "student involvement" language, there have been curricular materials and programs designed to promote student involvement. Although such resources do not focus exclusively on assessment, they will be integral components of efforts to actively involve students in transition planning and assessment. Space restrictions allow only brief descriptions of several such resources. A complete discussion of promoting student involvement is available from Wehmeyer and Sands (1998).

ChoiceMaker Self-Determination Transition Curriculum and Program

The ChoiceMaker Self-Determination Transition Curriculum (Martin & Marshall, 1995) consists of three sections: choosing goals, expressing goals, and taking action. Each section contains from two to four teaching goals and numerous teaching objectives addressing six transition areas. Included are an assessment tool, Choosing Goals lessons, the Self-Directed IEP, and Taking Action lessons. The program also includes a criterion-referenced self-determination transition assessment tool that matches the curricular sections. Specifically, the Self-Directed IEP lessons enable students to learn the leadership skills necessary to manage their IEP meeting and publicly disclose their interests, skills, limits, and goals identified through the Choosing Goals lessons. Rather than be passive participants at their IEP meetings, students learn to lead their meetings to the greatest extent of their ability. Table 3.1 lists the 11 steps students are taught.

Whose Future Is It Anyway?: A Student-Directed Transition Planning Program

Whose Future Is It Anyway? (Wehmeyer & Lawrence, 1995) consists of 36 sessions introducing students to the concept of transition and transition planning and enabling students to self-direct instruction related to 1) self- and disability awareness;

Table 3.1. Eleven steps for transition planning from the ChoiceMaker Self-Determination Transition Curriculum

1. Begin the meeting by stating the purpose.
2. Introduce everyone.
3. Review past goals and performance.
4. Ask for others' feedback.
5. State your school and transition goals.
6. Ask questions if you don't understand.
7. Deal with differences in opinion.
8. State the support you will need.
9. Summarize your goals.
10. Close the meeting by thanking everyone.
11. Work on individualized education program goals all year.

From "Choicemaker: A Self-Determination Transition Program" by J.E. Martin and L.H. Marshall, 1995, Intervention in School and Clinic, 30, 147–156. Copyright (1995) by PRO-ED, Inc. Reprinted with permission.

2) making decisions about transition-related outcomes; 3) identifying and securing community resources to support transition services; 4) writing and evaluating transition goals and objectives; 5) communicating effectively in small groups; and 6) developing skills to become an effective team member, leader, or self-advocate.

The materials are student-directed in that they are written for students as end-users. The level of support needed by students to complete activities varies a great deal, though the materials make every effort to ensure that students retain control while receiving the support they need to succeed. For example, although there is a coach's guide (Wehmeyer & Lawrence, 1995) to assist teachers in providing support, the identification of the person to serve as coach is left to the student. Students are instructed to identify a teacher or other person to serve as a coach and to take the coach's guide to that person.

Section I (titled "Getting to Know You") introduces the concept of transition and educational planning, provides information about transition requirements in IDEA, and enables students to identify who has attended past planning meetings, who is required to be present at meetings, and who they want involved in their planning process. Later, they are introduced to four transition outcome areas (employment, community living, postsecondary education, and recreation and leisure). Activities throughout the process focus on these transition outcomes.

In the second section (named "Making Decisions"), students learn a simple problem-solving process called DO IT! (see Table 3.2) by working through each step in the process to make a decision about a potential living arrangement, and then apply the process to make decisions about the three other transition outcome areas. The third section (called "How to Get What You Need, Sec. 101") enables students to locate community resources identified in previous planning meetings that are intended to provide supports in each of the transition outcome areas. Section

Table 3.2. DO IT! problem-solving strategy from Whose Future Is It Anyway?

D	Define the problem.
O	Outline your options.
I	Identify the outcome of each option.
T	Take action.
!	Get excited!

IV (titled "Goals, Objectives and the Future") enables learners to apply a set of rules to identify transition-related goals and objectives that are currently on their IEP or transition planning form, evaluate these goals based on their own transition interests and abilities, and develop additional goals to take to their next planning meeting. Students learn what goals and objectives are, how they should be written, and ways to track progress on goals and objectives.

The fifth section (called "Communication") introduces effective communication strategies for small group situations, like transition planning meetings. Students work through sessions that introduce different types of communication (verbal, body language, and so forth) and how to interpret these communicative behaviors, the differences between aggressive and assertive communication, how to effectively negotiate and compromise, when to use persuasion, and other skills that will enable them to be more effective communicators during transition planning meetings. The sixth and final session (called "Thank You, Honorable Chairperson") enables students to learn types and purposes of meetings, steps to holding effective meetings, and roles of the meeting chairperson and team members. Students are encouraged to work with school-district personnel to take a meaningful role in planning for and participating in the meeting, including eventually chairing a transition planning meeting.

Next S.T.E.P. (Student Transition and Educational Planning)

A third student-directed transition planning program is the Next S.T.E.P. curriculum (Halpern, et al., 1997). The two main purposes of this curriculum are to "teach students the skills they need to do transition planning" and to "engage students successfully in this process" (Halpern et al., 1997, p. 1). The curriculum uses videotape and print materials developed for specific audiences (students, teachers, family members) to help students engage in transition planning, self-evaluate transition needs, identify and select transition goals and activities, assume responsibility for conducting their own transition planning meeting, and monitor the implementation of their transition plans.

The curriculum consists of 16 lessons, clustered into four instructional units designed to be delivered in a 50-minute class period. These lessons include teacher and student materials, videos, guidelines for involving parents and family members, and a process for tracking student progress. Unit 1 (called "Getting Started") introduces and gives an overview of transition planning and is intended to enable students to understand the transition planning process and to motivate them to participate.

Unit 2 (named "Self-Exploration and Self-Evaluation") includes six lessons that focus on student self-evaluation. Students work through activities that identify unique interests, strengths, and weaknesses in various adult-outcome oriented areas. At the end of this unit, students complete the student form of the Transition Skills Inventory, mentioned previously. The student's self-evaluation of these areas are combined with similar evaluations by his or her teacher and a family member to form a basis for future transition planning activities.

Unit 3 (titled "Developing Goals and Activities") includes five lessons regarding transition goal identification in the four areas comprising the Transition Skills Inventory. Students identify their hopes and dreams, then select from a broad range of potential goals in each area, narrowing the total set of transition goals to four or five goals that they prefer. In addition, students choose activities that will help them pursue the goals they have selected. Unit 4 (named "Putting a Plan into Place") includes three lessons to prepare students for their transition planning meeting. The lessons emphasize the implementation of their plan and work with students to ensure that they monitor their progress and, if necessary, make adjustments.

Self-Advocacy Strategy for Education and Transition Planning

Van Reusen, Bos, Schumaker, and Deshler (1994) developed a procedure, the Self-Advocacy Strategy for Education and Transition Planning, that incorporates both types of strategies: student-directed transition planning and self-advocacy instruction. The program stresses the importance of self-advocacy to enhance student motivation and is "designed to enable students to systematically gain a sense of control and influence over their own learning and development" (Van Reusen et al., 1994, p. 1). Students progress through a series of lesson plans focusing on seven instructional stages. Stage 1 (titled "Orient and Make Commitments") broadly introduces education and transition planning meetings, the program itself, and how participation can increase student power and control in this process. Stage 2 (named "Describe") defines and provides detailed information about transition meetings and advantages students experience if they participate. In this stage the I PLAN steps of student participation are introduced. These steps, listed in Table 3.3., pro-

Table 3.3. I PLAN steps for a successful transition meeting

I	Inventory your strengths, areas to improve or learn, goals, and choices for learning or accommodations.
P	Provide your inventory information.
L	Listen and respond.
A	Ask questions.
N	Name your goals.

vide a simple algorithm that students can use to chart their participation in planning meetings.

In Stage 3 (called "Model and Prepare"), the teacher models the I PLAN steps so that students can see the process in action. Students complete an inventory (Step 1 in the I PLAN process) resulting in information that they can use at their conference. During Stage 4 (named "Verbal Practice"), in which students are asked question to make sure they know what to do during each step of the I PLAN strategy, and students then verbally rehearse each of the steps. In Stage 5 (titled "Group Practice and Feedback"), once students have demonstrated mastery of the steps in I PLAN, they participate in a simulated group conference. The student receives feedback from the teacher and other students, and the group generates suggestions on where the student needs improvement.

Stage 6 (called "Individual Practice and Feedback") allows the student to meet independently with the teacher for practice, feedback, and eventually mastery. The audio- or videotape from the previous stage is reviewed, and students provide a self-evaluation of their performance. The student and instructor work together to improve areas of self-identified need and engage in another simulated conference, which is also audio- or videotaped and used to document improvement and to reevaluate performance. Stage 7 (named "Generalization") is intended to generalize the I PLAN strategy to actual conferences. This stage has three phases: 1) preparing for and conducting the planning conference, 2) preparing for other uses of the strategy, and 3) preparing for subsequent conferences. Van Reusen and Bos (1990, 1994) have shown that the I PLAN strategy can be successfully implemented with students with disabilities, and its use results in increased motivation and participation.

Goal Action Planning

Turnbull and colleagues (1996) developed the Goal Action Planning procedure to enable youth with severe mental retardation and developmental disabilities to become involved in their educational planning. Goal Action Planning incorporates strategies from futures planning models to achieve this end. Students, family members, professionals, and others complete a process to identify goals, resources, and obstacles to achieving the student's desired outcomes. This process begins with the student's dreams and hopes. Using information gathered from the process, the student with a disability, supported by the group, formulates action plans across eight areas of daily life: domestic, transportation, employment, financial, recreational, social relationships, behavioral, and community participation.

SUMMARY

Assessment in self-determination and to determine student interests and preferences is, both legally and programmatically, an important component of the transition planning process; however, such efforts need to be accomplished within the context of empowerment evaluation framework where the unambiguous intent is to empower the student and better enable him or her to self-direct not only assessment but also involvement in transition planning. The various means to promote student involvement in transition planning, or similar processes, will be critical to such success as well.

REFERENCES

Clark, G.M. (1996). Transition planning assessment for secondary-level students with learning disabilities. In J.R. Patton & G. Blalock (Eds.), *Transition and students with learning disabilities: Facilitating the movement from school to adult life* (pp. 131–156). Austin, TX: PRO-ED.

Education for All Handicapped Children Act of 1975 , PL 94-142, 20 U.S.C. §§ 1400 *et seq.*

Fetterman, D.M. (1996). Empowerment evaluation: An introduction to theory and practice. In D.M. Fetterman, S.J. Kaftarian, & A. Wandersman (Eds.), *Empowerment evaluation: Knowledge and tools for self-assessment and accountability* (pp. 3–46). Thousand Oaks, CA: Sage Publications.

Field, S., & Hoffman, A. (1996). *Steps to Self-Determination: A Curriculum to Help Adolescents Learn to Achieve Their Goals.* Austin, TX: PRO-ED.

Gillespie, E.B., & Turnbull, A.P. (1983). It's my IEP!: Involving students in the planning process. *Teaching Exceptional Children, 29,* 27–29.

Halpern, A.S., Herr, C.M., Wolf, N.K., Lawson, J.D., Doren, B., & Johnson, M.D. (1997). *Next S.T.E.P.: Student Transition and Educational Planning. Teacher manual.* Eugene: University of Oregon.

Hughes, C., Pitkin, S.E., & Lorden, S.W. (1998). Assessing preferences and choices of persons with severe and profound disabilities. *Education and Training in Mental Retardation and Developmental Disabilities, 33,* 299–316.

Individuals with Disabilities Education Act (IDEA) Amendments of 1997, PL 105-17, 20 U.S.C. §§ 1400 *et seq.*

Kennedy, C., & Haring, T. (1993). Teaching choice making during social interactions to students with profound multiple disabilities. *Journal of Applied Behavior Analysis, 26,* 63–76.

Lewis, K., & Taymans, J.M. (1992). An examination of autonomous functioning skills of adolescents with learning disabilities. *Career Development for Exceptional Individuals, 15,* 37–46.

Martin, J.E., & Marshall, L.H. (1995). ChoiceMaker: A comprehensive self-determination transition program. *Intervention in School and Clinic, 30,* 147–156.

Martin, J.E., & Marshall, L.H. (1996). *ChoiceMaker Self-Determination Transition Assessment.* Longmont, CO: Sopris West.

Sigafoos, A.D., Feinstein, C.B., Damond, M., & Reiss, D. (1988). The measurement of behavioral autonomy in adolescence: The Autonomous Functioning Checklist. In C.B. Feinstein, A. Esman, J. Looney, G. Orvin, J. Schimel, A. Schwartzberg, A. Sorsky, & M. Sugar (Eds.), *Adolescent psychiatry* (Vol. 15, pp. 432–462). Chicago: University of Chicago Press.

Turnbull, A.P., Blue-Banning, M.J., Anderson, E.L., Turnbull, H.R., Seaton, K.A., & Dinas, P.A. (1996). Enhancing self-determination through group action planning: A holistic emphasis. In D.J. Sands & M.L. Wehmeyer (Eds.), *Self-determination across the life span: Independence and choice for people with disabilities* (pp. 237–256). Baltimore: Paul H. Brookes Publishing Co.

Van Reusen, A.K., & Bos, C.S. (1990). I PLAN: Helping students communicate in planning conferences. *Teaching Exceptional Children, 22*(4), 30–32.

Van Reusen, A.K., & Bos, C.S. (1994). Facilitating student participation in individualized education programs through motivation strategy instruction. *Exceptional Children, 60,* 466–475.

Van Reusen, A.K., Bos, C.S., Schumaker, J.B., & Deshler, D.D. (1994). *The Self-Advocacy Strategy for Education and Transition Planning.* Lawrence, KS: Edge Enterprises.

Wacker, D., Berg, W., Wiggins, B., Muldoon, M., & Cavanaugh, J. (1985). Evaluation of reinforcer preference for profoundly handicapped students. *Journal of Applied Behavior Analysis, 18,* 173–178.

Walker, J.H., & Shaw, S.F. (1995, October). *Perceptions of team members regarding the involvement of students with learning disabilities in transition planning.* Paper presented at the International Conference of the Division on Career Development and Transition, Raleigh, NC.

Wehmeyer, M.L., Agran, M., & Hughes, C. (1998). *Teaching self-determination to students with disabilities: Basic skills for successful transition.* Baltimore: Paul H. Brookes Publishing Co.

Wehmeyer, M.L., & Bolding, N. (1999). Self-determination across living and working environments: A matched-samples study of adults with mental retardation. *Mental Retardation, 37,* 353–363.

Wehmeyer, M.L., & Bolding, N. (in press). Enhanced self-determination of adults with intellectual disability as an outcome of moving to community-based work or living environments. *Journal of Intellectual Disability Research.*

Wehmeyer, M.L., & Kelchner, K. (1995). *The Arc's Self-Determination Scale.* Arlington, TX: The Arc National Headquarters.

Wehmeyer, M.L., Kelchner, K., & Richards, S. (1996). Essential characteristics of self-determined behavior in individuals with mental retardation. *American Journal of Mental Retardation, 100,* 632–642.

Wehmeyer, M.L., & Lawrence, M. (1995). Whose Future Is It Anyway?: Promoting student involvement in transition planning. *Career Development for Exceptional Individuals, 18,* 69–83.

Wehmeyer, M.L., Palmer, S.B., Agran, M., Mithaug, D., & Martin, J. (2000). Promoting causal agency: The Self-Determined Learning Model of Instruction. *Exceptional Children, 66,* 439–453.

Wehmeyer, M.L., & Sands, D.J. (1998). *Making it happen: Student involvement in education planning, decision-making, and instruction.* Baltimore: Paul H. Brookes Publishing Co.

Wehmeyer, M.L., & Schwartz, M. (1997). Self-determination and positive adult outcomes: A follow-up study of youth with mental retardation or learning disabilities. *Exceptional Children, 63,* 245–255.

Wehmeyer, M.L., & Schwartz, M. (1998). The relationship between self-determination, quality of life, and life satisfaction for adults with mental retardation. *Education and Training in Mental Retardation and Developmental Disabilities, 33,* 3–12.

Wolman, J.M., Campeau, P.L, DuBois, P.A., Mithaug, D.E., & Stolarski, V.S. (1994). *AIR Self-Determination Scale and user guide.* Stanford, CA: American Institute on Research.

4

The Three C's of Family Involvement
Things I Wish I Had Known

Barbara Buswell and Caren L. Sax

WILSON'S LATEST CHALLENGE

Barb's son, Wilson, had only a few months left before his official exit from the school district. The planning had been going on for a few years; he was steadily narrowing the focus of what steps he needed to take to get him going in the right direction—specifically, attending college. Wilson had always liked school. Academic policies and politics fascinated him, especially when he was investigating how they both helped and hindered his own progress. His family was behind him 100% and eager to help him pursue his dreams while they struggled to create and maintain the necessary supports. Unfortunately, it seemed that the responsibility for organizing planning meetings typically fell on them.

A meeting was called to urge everyone to "think outside the box." Wilson, two peers who provided support for him, the transition teacher, the representative from the supported living agency, and Barb attended the meeting that was facilitated by Caren. Of note, those who did not attend included the vocational rehabilitation counselor and representatives from both the community college that Wilson had been attending and the university to which he had applied. Wilson's former employer from a summer camp was on the guest list the family compiled; however, for some reason she was not invited.

The handling of the guest list was indicative of the communication difficulties that had plagued Wilson's team for the past 2 years. The services didn't seem to fit Wilson's characteristics. The traditional support needs seemed to be too great for professionals who were unfamiliar with someone who communicated in such nontraditional ways. There seemed to be a lack of experience in trying to design a plan for Wilson and an assumption that there was someone else out there who knew how to do it better. Why does the transition process break down when dealing with youth like Wilson? People said that transition would be hard, but does it really need to be this difficult?

CLEARING A PATH

Over the years, Barb has shared stories of Wilson as he experienced everything from family rafting trips, to inclusive elementary and high schools, to his first political initiation in Washington, D.C. (Buswell, 1999). Throughout his life, his family has challenged the status quo, maintaining high expectations despite the significant challenges that he faces physically, communicatively, and medically. As they approached the end of his high school career and began considering options for adulthood, they have encountered unexpected challenges. They have also made some important realizations to share with other families as they clear a path through the transition process.

Transition planning can be overwhelming—especially when dealing with unfamiliar adult disability service delivery systems. Familiarity with the public school system does not necessarily prepare families to deal effectively with these new bureaucracies. Families need to learn different terminology as well as new ways of doing business (San Diego State University, 2000). In order to ease some of the mystery about the process, this chapter provides essential information and a collection of tools for families and educators. As key stakeholders in the futures of their sons and daughters, families must be equal participants in the decision-making and planning processes.

Research and personal stories suggest that families experience greater success in advocating when they create a deliberate process to pass along what they have learned from year to year; from team to team; and from school to adult agencies, worksites, and college campuses. The biggest challenge when leaving the school system, where families typically communicate with one instructional team, is moving to the community with multiple points of contact (e.g., job coaches, college instructors, co-workers, supervisors, agency directors). Coordinating and communicating with these multiple players in the adult world often causes considerable confusion for families. We have outlined some processes to help families maintain instructional and support practices and strategies that work for a particular individual and eliminate those that do not. We have organized our ideas according to three C's: credibility, continuity, and conscientiousness. Wilson has taught us all a great deal about change and flexibility through the phases of his life. We hope that the following realizations will help other families plan more proactively for the adult lives of individuals with disabilities.

CREDIBILITY

Family members must establish credibility in at least two ways. First, they must clearly understand the legal processes and procedures that guide service delivery in special education and transition services (see Seyler & Buswell, 2001, for specific information about the individualized education program [IEP] process). Then, they must establish positive relationships with professionals who work within the system. Let's explore how each of these components adds to a family's credibility.

In order to participate effectively, parents need to understand their rights and responsibilities under the Individuals with Disabilities Education Act (IDEA) of 1990, PL 101-476, which was reauthorized by Congress as the IDEA Amendments of 1997 (PL 105-17). This law provides students with disabilities the right to a free appropriate public education (FAPE). Providing an appropriate education also means educating students with disabilities in the least restrictive environment (LRE). This means students with disabilities learn in general education classrooms alongside their peers who do not have disabilities, when appropriate, and that schools provide supplementary aids and services to support students with disabilities to be successful in general education classrooms (Fisher, Sax, & Pumpian, 1999).

Contacting the Parent Training and Information Center in your state via the Technical Assistance Alliance for Parent Centers (http://www.taalliance.org) or the U.S. Department of Education (http://www.ed.gov/offices/OSERS/OSEP) for more information about education laws and family rights is extremely important. The U.S. Department of Education's Office of Special Education and Rehabilitative Services has developed an IEP guide (http://www.ed.gov/offices/OSERS/OSEP/IEP_Guide), which explains roles, responsibilities, and guidelines in jargon-free language. It is important to know the intent of the legislation in order to speak with credibility about the related issues. The sections of this web site that address transition from school to adult life are based on IDEA's "Statement of Transition Service Needs":

> The IEP must include . . . [f]or each student with a disability beginning at age 14 (or younger, if determined appropriate by the IEP team), and updated annually, a statement of the transition service needs of the student under the applicable components of the student's IEP that focuses on the student's courses of study (such as participation in advanced-placement courses or a vocational education program). (34 CFR §300.347[b][1])

According to the regulations, transition refers to activities designed to prepare students with disabilities for adult life. This may include developing postsecondary education and career goals; obtaining work experience while in school; setting up linkages with adult service providers such as the vocational rehabilitation agency; and whatever might be appropriate for the student, given his or her interests, preferences, skills, and needs. All students need to begin to plan for their futures as they enter high school and continue to evaluate and further modify those plans as they near the age of exit. Planning for transition at age 14 (or younger if found appropriate by the IEP team) includes helping the student select classes and other activities that will lead to his or her postschool goals. Transition services beginning at age 16 involve providing the student with a coordinated set of services to help ease the move from school to adult life. Services focus on tapping the student's needs or interests in such areas as higher education or training, employment, adult services, independent living, or taking part in the community. It is important to not limit the possibilities for the student's and his or her family's dreams for the future to be a fully participating and included member of the high school and later, the adult community (Tashie, Malloy, & Lichtenstein, 1998).

IDEA '97 allows for students with disabilities to be served by their school district until the age of 21, or in some states older; however, students with disabilities usually participate in high school graduation with their classmates who do not have IEPs. (In order to continue to serve the student, however, schools then hold the official diploma until the student exits the school system at age 21.) After graduation, transition services for 18- to 21-year-old students are provided in community, school, and work environments.

In states that transfer rights at the age of majority (age 18), the IEP must include a statement that the student has been informed of any rights that will transfer to him or her at least 1 year before the student comes of age. This means that students make their own decisions, including agreements about postsecondary education. In the states where this happens, disability-related information is confidential and must come from the student. It is important for parents to keep informed about research on current best practices and effective ways to best help students learn. Also, parents need to learn how and when to speak up and what to do when the process is not working.

In addition to understanding the planning processes, parents must also develop credibility with the professionals who will interact with their family members. Right or wrong, documentation that is developed collaboratively between families and professionals is often given more consideration than information offered solely by families. It is essential that transition teachers or special education advocates/teachers work together with families in order to record successful and unsuccessful support and instructional strategies. Parents are valuable sources of information; however, the way in which that information is presented can either increase or diminish the parents' credibility. For example, if the family and student have expressed interest in pursuing postsecondary education and the transition teacher describes only vocational opportunities, the focus on continuing education may be viewed as unrealistic by adult services providers. If the expectations, goals, modifications, and accommodations are recorded consistently, the credibility level increases. There are too many stories reported by families labeled troublesome or demanding simply because they wanted to see their adult sons and daughters have the opportunity for an inclusive and quality adult life. As more students experience inclusive education in kindergarten through grade 12, they are expecting, and in some cases demanding, that their lives as adults continue to be filled with inclusive activities in natural environments and with meaningful relationships.

CONTINUITY

The second C refers to continuity. Figuring out ways for families, school personnel, and adult agency professionals to work together to establish and maintain continuity for students as they leave high school is challenging at best. As with transitions during the school years (e.g., from elementary to middle school, from middle to high school), too often the key personnel must start over in learning how to provide the most appropriate supports to a student, particularly to those with significant disabilities. Trial and error takes precious time away from addressing new goals in new environments. Although cumulative records accompany students, sometimes the most essential information learned by previous instructional and support teams does not transfer easily into documents. Challenges that were once overcome are often faced again. If the new team from the adult agency staff does not know the individual, that student may lose motivation, parents may become upset, and people on the new team may begin questioning why this student has been accepted into their agency. Furthermore, if agency staff are not familiar with this person's strengths, needs, and interests, they may not be effective advocates in identifying new work or educational environments.

This lack of experience, information, and/or training on how to teach or support a person with a particular disability leaves employers and college instructors frustrated. Without proactive planning and effective communication, individuals may become vulnerable. The intentional transfer of knowledge, information, and support is critical to prevent reactive situations from occurring. How many times have you heard, "I wish someone could just send the right information so we don't have to reinvent the wheel?" Then, service providers proceed to not only reinvent the wheel but to reinvent the axle, body, transmission, and sometimes, the whole car!

Roadblocks for Continuity

Why does transition seem so complicated? First, a variety of service delivery and support paradigms exist in different systems (e.g., public schools, developmental disabilities, rehabilitation, postsecondary institutions). Often a student who has been successful in one environment encounters a new way of being provided resources and supports in other places. Unfortunately, the change is not always for the better. Second, supporting students in natural environments requires individualized and unique support approaches. These approaches may change from year to year, and what may work for one team may not be successful for another.

A third complication in the transition process can be attributed to inadequate (or nonexistent) in-service training and technical assistance or consultation for adult agency providers. Staff need immediate information and strategies during the first few weeks of the transition when personnel are typically very busy and resources are not easily accessible or available. If professionals with the time and expertise are not available to assist or be proactive, individuals with disabilities suffer. No one feels ownership or responsibility for their programming or support, and at that point, few are likely to volunteer to come forth. Consequently, as parents watch their children flounder after having had a successful experience in a previous environment, they become frustrated. In response, many feel forced to take the issue to a higher administrative or judicial level and risk being labeled as pushy and adversarial.

As a result, parents turn to the IEP and individualized transition plan (ITP) as compliance tools, rather than as a road map for the student's individualized support. In the end, families are in conflict with various support agencies, and the very approach that would help is sabotaged. Most parents prefer to work collaboratively with the team to support their child, but many feel that this route is impossible when they are forced to compromise their situation or expectations because of service delivery practices that do not work. Furthermore, when transition assessment and planning is being approached for one student at a time, rather than in a broad systemic way, each family must fight its own battle, leaving little changed for families who follow. Strategies for addressing these systemic issues are covered in more detail in Chapter 9.

Strategies for Success

What strategies can be used to ensure continuity for students with significant disabilities as they enter adult life? The most effective strategies are implemented simultaneously both top–down (i.e., used by adult agency administrators) as well as bottom–up (i.e., used by school personnel who send the student to the new situation, the adult agency staff who will receive the student, and the student and family.)

Strategies for the sending and receiving teams that have formed around an individual student include thoughtful planning and an expectation that the planning will be implemented. Each team develops a plan of what needs to be accomplished and by when. While the end of a school year is hectic, at best, planning must be initiated before the public school year ends. The sending team should document approaches and strategies that have worked well in supporting the student. In addition, they can interview and document information from key people who supported the student successfully or who understood the strategies that created the student successes. Whether they record this information on audiotape, videotape, or in notebooks with photographs, it is essential for them to have input from classroom teachers, specialists, and classmates of the student. A further helpful step is to make an opportunity available with the sending and receiving team members to share information on how the individual responds in different situations. Finally, one of the richest information resources is the expertise and knowledge of the student's family.

Families

Families can be instrumental in developing a record of successful strategies for the new adult support team to consult when they get stuck. One way to do this is to create a transition portfolio. A transition portfolio can be a document for people to learn about critical strengths-based information as well as supports that work. It can also be a training tool. If the team decides to create a transition portfolio, there are some essential components to include and a number of pitfalls to avoid. Transition portfolios should include the following kinds of information learned from the school experience:

1. Descriptions of the student that are positive

2. A student profile describing the student's strengths, interests, favorite activities, IEP/ITP goals or learning priorities for the year, as well as other unique information that services providers need to know

3. A list of tasks that a teacher assistant or a paraprofessional completed that defined their roles in relation to the student and to the teacher. In addition, some families have included the job posting for a paraprofessional position used at school. These often describe the personal qualities desired by the student and the family and could be used to identify effective personal support providers in the future.

4. Pointers about physical assistance that the student has needed

5. Tips on communicating with the student, particularly if the student has difficulty expressing him- or herself or if the people around the student have difficulty understanding. These may include videotaped segments demonstrating a conversation with use of picture communication symbols or augmentative and alternative communication devices.

6. Behavioral supports that work, a description of situations to avoid or ways to structure situations to eliminate behavior challenges for the student

7. Ways to involve the student in different classroom activities across subject areas (e.g., math, English, science) and instructional strategies (e.g., small-group work, lectures, individual work) for consideration in future educational environments such as college or adult school. Entries in this area should include samples of the student's work including the original class assignment, a description of adaptations or modifications to classroom activities and assignments, and informal and formal accommodations used in test taking or classroom presentations.

8. Unique environmental arrangements that help support the student and other unique dimensions of the student's support plan, such as seating and positioning needs, personal care details, noise level tolerance, lighting, and climate comfort levels

9. Descriptions of the team planning processes, such as when the team met and how members communicated and collaborated. Though the receiving team is likely to work differently, teams generally report that it is helpful to understand the routines of the previous team.

10. Description of any equipment, devices, or other assistive technology that a student uses, and how it is accessed, used, mounted, stored, transferred, and so forth as well as the names of resource people in this area for maintenance and repairs.

We give you one caution: Transition portfolios should NOT be the only, or the primary, mode for transferring information about the individual with a disability from a sending team to a receiving team. In addition, the following pitfalls should be avoided.

1. Do not limit the description of the student to problems, troubles, or weaknesses.

2. Avoid using descriptors that could limit opportunities for this student or discourage people from getting to know him or her directly.

3. Discourage readers from assuming that they know or understand this person just because they read this portfolio.

CONSCIENTIOUSNESS

Families must be conscientious about the day-to-day details while ensuring access to natural environments and activities. In my life, I must help Wilson to remember his transportation times, finish his college homework, and take enough food for the amount of time he will be away from home. While our family attends to these details, we cannot lose sight of our goals—success in college, good friends, and real employment.

Much of the information in Wilson's transition portfolio focuses on him and his unique strengths and needs. While individual assessments and portfolios are critical, we must also assess more than just the person. We must assess the supports and environments that are being considered. In order to evaluate potential community environments (e.g., work, college, recreation, living situations), students and families may want to visit community sites where adult agencies are providing supports to an individual with disabilities. It is essential to prearrange the visit through agency staff well in advance so that meetings between employment and/or instructional personnel and families may take place with minimal disruption and site visits may be well-organized. A productive visit takes good planning. When visiting a worksite, it is important to be mindful of visitation etiquette. Here are some helpful tips when visiting a place of employment:

- Try to schedule your time so as to be as nonintrusive as possible. Schedule the time through agency personnel so as to arrive at times when the most relevant activities may be observed.

- Schedule meetings with potential employers and co-workers throughout the day at times convenient to them. Be respectful of everyone's time during these meetings.

- Before the visit, become thoroughly familiar with the questions you have decided to explore. Discuss them with agency personnel in order to include all important issues.

- During conversation times—such as during breaks or lunch, walks through work areas, or meetings with the staff—be ready to ask questions that you noted during observation sessions. Use these occasions to ask for greater clarification about the work culture and philosophy of the business.

- Remember that everything about a site reflects the way it is intentionally or unintentionally supporting all of its employees. Look at things such as maintenance of the building and grounds, accessibility, menus in the cafeteria, workplace and office décor, lighting, ventilation, noise levels, office placement, and ambiance of the break room.

- Ask first before taking pictures. Cameras can be a distraction, and in some cases, it is against the law or company policy to take pictures without permission.

- Notetaking can also be a distraction. It is always best to ask if unsure, although it is sometimes easier to observe and then jot down notes after leaving.

- Remember, you are a guest who has been invited to share in a different organizational dynamic than what you may have been familiar with in schools. Your very presence changes what typically happens, regardless of how accustomed the agency or business is to hosting visitors. As much as possible, be a gracious, appreciative observer.

Many of these same tips may be applied to visiting other sites, including community colleges or universities, recreational facilities, and volunteer opportunities at nonprofit associations. Consideration of details must extend to transportation, finances, health care, and benefits—the same issues that everyone entering adulthood must contemplate (Weinberg, 1996). The main points to remember are to plan ahead, organize your purposes for the visit, and remain open to observing different procedures and organizations without judgment or criticism.

Another tool which can be used to find out how the agency, worksite, or postsecondary educational institution is presently doing is the Integration Quotient (IQ) questionnaire. When exploring the world of adult services providers, it is important to assess the match between your family's expectations and the agency's ability to meet those needs. This resource is a list of questions adapted from the Minnesota Governor's Planning Council on Developmental Disabilities (see http://www.ici.umn.edu for more information) to use when considering adult services delivery systems (see Figure 4.1). These questions were designed to assist families and students with disabilities to assess the level of integration efforts of a particular agency or service delivery system. They can also help to show areas where the agency has made strides in the right direction and target areas that still need improvement.

CONSTANCY AND CREATIVITY

Persistence, endurance, tenacity, and determination are all synonyms for constancy, the C that families insist is the most important. Finding that energy within as well as from friends and relatives helps to ensure that individuals with disabilities have the opportunities that all children deserve. Many professionals in the public education or adult services systems have family members with disabilities and are familiar with the issues and frustrations. Make them your allies and help to change the system by starting a discourse on collaboration rather than on turf issues. Keep the unwavering focus on the accomplishments, interests, and dreams of your sons and daughters. And, above all, be creative by thinking outside the box while holding on to your dreams (Buswell, Schaffner, & Seyler, 1999). These are the assessment data that count and that can help to reframe the system's view of challenges and barriers into opportunities and successes.

Administrative and Board of Directors Commitment

1. Has the agency administration taken a position emphasizing the ability of individuals with disabilities to live and work in integrated community environments?   YES   NO
   Notes:

2. Has the agency administration demonstrated leadership in promoting the community inclusion of individuals with disabilities through promotional materials, building accessibility, presentations, conferences, scheduling flexibility, or published vision and mission statements?   YES   NO
   Notes:

3. Have administrators, program managers, job developers, and other support staff received in-service training on inclusive community research, values, and practices (e.g., person-centered planning, natural supports, self-determination) during the past year?   YES   NO
   Notes:

Location and Transportation

4. Are individuals with disabilities employed in businesses within reasonable distances from their homes?   YES   NO
   Notes:

5. Do individuals with disabilities have access to activities in their neighborhoods or through the use of public transportation?   YES   NO
   Notes:

6. Do individuals with disabilities have access to the same transportation that they would if they did not have disabilities?   YES   NO
   Notes:

Time and Activities

7. Are the agency's schedules and staffing patterns enough to accomodate jobs, continuing education, or recreational activites of the individual's choice?   YES   NO
   Notes:

8. How much time do individuals with disabilities spend with people without disabilities? Specify amount of time _____.
   Circle environments that apply:

   WORK   TRANSPORTATION   RECREATION   VOLUNTEER WORK
   WORK BREAKS   LUNCH   SOCIAL ACTIVITIES   OTHER

   Notes:

9. Do individuals with disabilities receive support services in postsecondary settings with students who do not have disabilities?   YES   . NO
   Circle support services that apply:

   MODIFIED CURRICULUM   TESTING ACCOMMODATIONS   INTERPRETER SERVICES
   PEER SUPPORT OR MENTORING   SUPPORT STAFF   COMMUNICATION DEVICES
   ADAPTIVE EQUIPMENT   ASSISTIVE TECHNOLOGY   OTHER

   Notes:

Figure 4.1. Test the integration quotient of your future community. (Instructions: To answer these questions, you should speak to several people. In some cases, you may want to review written documents.)

REFERENCES

Buswell, B. (1999). Families: The key to continuity. In D. Fisher, C. Sax, & I. Pumpian (Eds.), *Inclusive high schools: Learning from contemporary classrooms* (pp. 171–181). Baltimore: Paul H. Brookes Publishing Co.

Buswell, B.E., Schaffner, C.B., & Seyler, A.B. (Eds.). (1999). *Opening doors: Connecting students to curriculum, classmates, and learning* (2nd ed.). Colorado Springs, CO: Peak Parent Center.

Fisher, D., Sax, C., & Pumpian, I. (1999). *Inclusive high schools: Learning from contemporary classrooms.* Baltimore: Paul H. Brookes Publishing Co.

Individuals with Disabilities Education Act (IDEA) of 1990, PL 101-476, 20 U.S.C. §§ 1400 *et seq.*

Individuals with Disabilities Education Act (IDEA) Amendments of 1997, PL 105-17, 20 U.S.C. §§ 1400 *et seq.*

San Diego State University. (2000). *Plan smart: Focus on the future and putting it all together to achieve a successful life.* San Diego: Author.

Seyler, A.B., & Buswell, B.E. (2001). *Individual education plans: Involved effective parents.* Colorado Springs, CO: Peak Parent Center.

Tashie, C., Malloy, J.M., & Lichtenstein, S.J. (1998). Transition or graduation?: Supporting all students to plan for the future. In C.M. Jorgensen, *Restructuring high schools for all students: Taking inclusion to the next level* (pp. 233–260). Baltimore: Paul H. Brookes Publishing Co.

Weinberg, C. (1996). *The transition guide for college juniors and seniors: How to prepare for the future.* New York: New York University Press.

5

Informal Assessment Procedures

Carolyn Hughes and Erik W. Carter

LUCINDA GETS A JOB

Spring semester was fast approaching, and Mr. Perez had to make a decision regarding Lucinda's first job placement. His students always worked at either the Inglewood Hotel, Lockeland Billing Center, or Edgefield Bakery, so it was really just a matter of deciding among them. He completed an adaptive behavior scale and found that Lucinda had social skill and language impairments that would prevent her from working at the hotel. After all, he didn't want guests feeling uncomfortable around her! Next, Mr. Perez administered a vocational aptitude test and discovered that Lucinda did not possess sufficient clerical skills for a job at a billing center. Finally, Mr. Perez had Lucinda complete a career inventory, where she scored highest in the area of food service. Based on his assessments, it was clear—Edgefield Bakery would be the best job placement for Lucinda.

Lucinda, however, had always wanted a job at the mall with her friends, so it surprised her when Mr. Perez told her she would be working at Edgefield Bakery. She had seen that place before! Everyone worked at a table by themselves stuffing loaves of bread in bags. Lucinda knew her endurance and coordination weren't that great. And fastening those tiny twist-ties—her fingers hurt just thinking about it. Moreover, the break room was on the second floor, and there was no elevator for her wheelchair. She had only pointed to those restaurant pictures because they showed lots of young people in them. No one at the bakery was anywhere near her age! Why hadn't anyone tried to figure out what she wanted to do?

FORMAL ASSESSMENT

In the past, practitioners often used formal assessment procedures to make instructional decisions by comparing a student's performance to a normative standard (Sitlington, 1996). For high school students with severe disabilities, however, formal assessment may not provide much information that is useful for transition planning (Clark, 1998). Using these procedures, practitioners may assess students in relation to a construct, such as *vocational ability,* which may have little relevance to students' immediate or future environments. Because formal assessment may not reflect the actual demands of a worksite or other environment, its predictive validity with respect to a student's future success may be limited (Agran & Morgan, 1991). In addition, valued outcomes, such as social relationships or community participation, may be difficult to measure using formal assessment procedures, particularly with students who may have limited language skills (Siegel-Causey & Allinder, 1998). If teachers rely exclusively on formal assessment, the outcomes may be similar to those experienced by Lucinda and Mr. Perez.

INFORMAL ASSESSMENT

Increasingly, transition assessment is characterized by informal assessment procedures (Sitlington, 1996). Like more formal assessment, informal assessment is a process for identifying a student's strengths, interests, preferences, and needs; however, the primary strength of informal assessment is its direct relevance to instructional planning and the design of educational supports. For example, informal assessment can be conducted in any environment in which a student is participating, allowing practitioners to identify skills and supports within the context of a specific environment (Rosenthal-Malek, 1998). In addition, informal assessment instruments can be developed or modified to focus on specific skills relevant to a student's daily life rather than generic traits or abilities (Macfarlane, 1998). Furthermore, informal assessment can be conducted by professionals, parents, employers, co-workers, peers, and even students themselves.

Examples of informal assessment include direct observation, interviews, student or parent surveys, ecological inventories, task analyses, and social support assessments. This chapter proposes an eight-step model for guiding transition teachers and other practitioners in 1) selecting appropriate informal assessments; 2) developing and modifying their own informal assessments; and 3) translating assessment information into individualized transition goals, objectives, and curricular plans. We begin by describing assumptions of the proposed model of assessment. Next, we provide an overview of the model and applications of each of its steps. We conclude with a case study illustrating application of the model in practice to guide teachers in its implementation.

ASSUMPTIONS OF THE PROPOSED MODEL

Our proposed assessment model is designed to guide practitioners in selecting and applying informal assessment procedures with transition-age students. This model is based on the following assumptions derived from research and practice.

Student Involvement

One purpose of transition assessment is to assist students in making meaningful decisions by becoming aware of their strengths, skills, interests, and preferences relative to opportunities and demands in the environment (Sitlington, Neubert, & Leconte, 1997). Informal assessments should be student centered, allowing students to participate in decisions regarding procedures to use, possible modifications, and interpretation and application of results (Smith et al., 1996). Increased student involvement may result in a more accurate representation of a student's strengths, interests, and needs (Macfarlane, 1998) and is clearly supported by the Individuals with Disabilities Education Act (IDEA) Amendments of 1997 (PL 105-17), which mandate student involvement in the development of educational programming. Therefore, the focus of informal assessment should be the individual student. Assessments should not be conducted simply because they are part of an established protocol of a high school program (Agran & Morgan, 1991). Furthermore, consistent with the philosophy and research supporting the IDEA Amendments of 1997, assessments should raise expectations for students by focusing on their *strengths* and strategies to *support* their education.

Student, Family, and Cultural Values

Transition assessment benefits from close communication and interaction between school personnel and students and their families. At the same time, high school students and their families are from increasingly diverse cultural backgrounds and hold increasingly diverse values. As affirmed by the IDEA Amendments of 1997, practitioners must be sensitive to the cultural values that influence students and their families. In conducting informal assessments, practitioners must remember that skills and supports being assessed are influenced by a student's cultural and family background (Lim & Browder, 1994).

Collaboration

The IDEA Amendments of 1997 call for active involvement of all stakeholders—students, family and community members, employers, co-workers, and practitioners—in the design, implementation, and interpretation of informal assessments (Sitlington, 1996). Through collaboration, multiple individuals are given the opportunity to share their unique perspectives and expertise concerning a student's strengths, support needs, and future plans and to assist in developing creative instructional strategies and supports (Rainforth & York-Barr, 1997). The input of family members is an especially critical component of transition assessment for students who are entering adult life in order to ensure that educational programs match students' and families' desired postschool outcomes (Thompson, Fulk, & Piercy, 2000).

Natural Environments

Traditional assessment may result in assumptions about what a student *cannot* do, limiting students' opportunities to participate in a range of everyday activities and environments (Rainforth & York-Barr, 1997). Consequently, it is essential that informal assessment take place in the actual environments in which students participate to determine what they *can* do and what supports will maximize their performance (Macfarlane, 1998). Moreover, because a student's strengths and needs will vary according to the demands of different environments, it is important to assess students in a variety of environments. Although practitioners have used simulated environments in the past, skills must be assessed in the environments they are expected to occur to determine if a skill actually has been acquired (Thurlow & Elliott, 1998).

Ongoing Assessment

Throughout a student's adolescent years, change should be expected: students' goals evolve, skills are mastered, need for support changes, and new environments are encountered. Information gathered at one point in a student's life may not accurately represent his or her situation later. Informal transition assessment must be an ongoing process carried out on a regular basis to ensure its validity (Sitlington et al., 1997).

OVERVIEW OF THE MODEL

To offer guidance in effectively conducting informal transition assessment, we propose a model that assists practitioners in 1) choosing appropriate assessment procedures and instruments, 2) modifying existing assessments or developing new ones, and 3) using assessment information to develop transition goals and make instructional and curricular decisions. This model is based on research and recommended practice in secondary transition and is composed of eight steps (see Table 5.1). This section describes the steps of the model with examples of application.

Step 1: Determine the Purpose of Assessment

The first step in conducting informal assessment is to determine the purpose for assessment. For example, a transition teacher may wish to know how well a student is being accepted into a worksite or general education classroom environment, or a parent may want to know what jobs are available in the neighborhood that match her son's interests. The aspects of a student's life and educational experiences that could be a focus of assessment are unlimited—social skills, career interests, choice-making skills, environmental supports, or opportunities for community involvement. For example, Benz, Lindstorm, and Yovanoff (2000) asked high school students to identify the factors they believed were most valuable in helping them achieve their transition goals. Common themes identified by students included individualized services and personalized attention from staff.

The type of information needed for making decisions about a student's current and future experiences should guide informal assessments (Sitlington et al., 1997). Informal assessments can address three primary areas: the student, the environment, and the educational program.

Table 5.1. Steps of the Informal Transition Assessment Model

1. Determine the purpose of assessment.
2. Identify relevant behaviors and environments.
3. Verify Steps 1 and 2 based on input from student and important others.
4. Choose appropriate assessment procedures.
5. Modify procedures as needed.
6. Conduct the assessment.
7. Use assessment findings to identify transition goals and objectives.
8. Develop curricular plans to achieve goals.

Assessing Students

Effective educational planning and decision making are the product of collecting and analyzing relevant information. Decisions regarding areas in which to focus instruction and develop supports must be based on information that is relevant to a student's progress (Macfarlane, 1998). Questions about a student that informal assessment may address include

- What school, work, and community environments is a student currently involved in or interested in becoming involved?
- What skills does a student have relative to those environments?
- Which of those skills need to be developed further?
- What do important others think about those skills?
- What additional information is needed about the student?

Assessing Environments

Practitioners are increasingly recognizing the impact that environmental factors have on a student's performance (Thurlow & Elliott, 1998). Students' performance can be influenced by such variables as employer or teacher expectations, variability in job tasks, peer support, and the physical arrangement of the environment. Assessing environmental factors can inform practitioners regarding the skills, knowledge, and supports that are critical to successful participation in an environment (Phelps & Hanley-Maxwell, 1997).

Assessing Programs

Informal assessment can also be used to determine the quality of transition services and supports being provided to students. Relevant questions may include

- How effective is a program in helping students achieve their current and future school, work, and community living goals?

- What program modifications or additions need to be made?
- What recommendations do stakeholders, including students and family members, have for improving the transition planning process (Vallecorsa, deBettencourt, & Garriss, 1992)?

Step 2: Identify Relevant Behaviors and Environments

After the purpose of an assessment has been established, the next step is to identify relevant behaviors to be assessed and corresponding environments in which assessment should be conducted. Behaviors and environments that are targeted should, of course, relate directly to the established purpose of the assessment. For example, if the extent to which a student is self-directed is of concern, a teacher may identify choice making, self-management, or decision making as appropriate behaviors for assessment. Reid, Parsons, and Green (1998) identified choice of work tasks as the target behavior when conducting work preference assessments for three employees with severe disabilities. Similarly, Farley and Johnson (1999) targeted vocational self-awareness, career decisiveness, job application performance, and job interview performance in an effort to assess career exploration and job-seeking skills of students with disabilities.

In addition, behaviors should be assessed within the environments in which they are expected to be performed. Campbell, Campbell, and Brady (1998) recommended identifying relevant current and future environments in a student's life when determining instructional curricula. Many behaviors are expected to be performed across more than one environment (e.g., choice making, self-management, social skills), whereas others may be relevant to a particular environment, such as grooming or cooking. Therefore, multiple environments should be targeted as the context for informal assessment. For example, choice making has been assessed in community environments (Cooper & Browder, 1998), worksites (Parsons, Reid, & Green, 1998), and residences (Newton, Ard, & Horner, 1993).

Step 3: Verify Steps 1 and 2 Based on Input from Student and Important Others

After identifying the purpose of the assessment and the behaviors and environments of primary interest, practitioners should verify these selections with students and important others. It is essential that decisions made about assessment, instruction, and planning represent the priorities and values of students and their families. In addition, input from other transition team members can help confirm the validity of decisions being made, as perceived by important others. For example, Mactavish, Mahon, and Lutfiyya (2000) interviewed individuals with intellectual disabilities regarding their perspectives on the meaning of social integration. Interviewees, it was found, viewed social integration differently than did researchers. Similarly, Park, Gonsier-Gerdin, Hoffman, Whaley, and Yount (1998) found that job coaches and teachers held different understandings of social relationships than did researchers. Researchers have also solicited the perspectives of teachers, parents, and students with respect to including students with severe disabilities in general education classes (Janney, Snell, Beers, & Raynes, 1995; Smith, 1997; York & Tundidor, 1995) and setting goals for social interaction (Hughes, Killian, & Fischer, 1996).

Step 4: Choose Appropriate Assessment Procedures

The decision to use a particular assessment procedure should be based on the purpose of the assessment, the behaviors and environments of concern, and input of important others. A variety of informal assessment procedures are available and selection should be based on the type of information needed (Ramasamy & Taylor, 1996). For example, teachers in five states identified assessment procedures (e.g., observations, interviews, surveys) that were appropriate for assessing students with severe disabilities across five curricular domains (Ysseldyke & Olsen, 1999). Hughes and colleagues (1999) used direct observation and comparative analysis to assess the extent to which students with mental retardation interacted with their general education peers.

In deciding which type of informal assessment procedure to use, practitioners should consider if the information needed would best be obtained by directly observing a behavior or environment or by taking indirect measures, such as interviewing parents or asking an employer to complete a written survey. For example, if the purpose of an assessment is to determine the extent to which a student interacts with co-workers on the job, direct observation may be the most appropriate procedure; however, and as emphasized in the IDEA Amendments of 1997, more than one assessment procedure may be needed to obtain necessary information. In the example of determining co-worker interaction at work, interviewing fellow employees and supervisors may indicate how well a student is accepted into workplace culture. Having the student complete a questionnaire may also reveal how comfortable he or she feels on the job. Examples of some informal transition assessment procedures that can be used to provide information about students, environments, or programs include direct observation; interviews; questionnaires, surveys, and checklists; interest inventories; self-assessments; social support assessments; and ecological inventories.

Direct Observation

Observing students' involvement in school, work, and community activities is a primary means of obtaining information about how a student is performing within a specific environment. Behavioral observations involve assessing aspects of a student's performance in everyday environments *as they actually occur.* Because many behaviors, such as greeting customers, have no permanent product (e.g., score on a written test), teachers or others must observe directly whether the behavior actually occurred. Behavioral observations also can enhance or confirm information gathered through other methods, such as parent surveys. In addition, they can be conducted across many environments, such as work or recreational sites, shopping malls, apartments, or community college campuses. Teachers can observe students and narratively record their actions and those of others (*narrative recording*) or they can tally specific behaviors a student performs during a fixed amount of time (*event recording*). In addition, a teacher can observe how long a behavior occurs during preset periods of time (*interval recording*) or how many steps a student performs in a sequence of behaviors required to complete a task (*task analysis*). Figure 5.1 shows an example of an event recording datasheet that can be used to observe multiple behaviors required for a student who is working in a department store.

Interviews

Interviews are valuable tools for determining how well a student is performing or how effective an instructional program is in terms of the expectations of important others. Perspectives can be obtained from a variety of people, such as family members, peers, co-workers, employers, teachers, and neighbors, as well as the students themselves. For example, Sacks, Wolffe, and Tierney (1998) interviewed parents of students with visual impairments about the students' academic involvement and participation in social, recreational, and work experiences. Socialization and career development were identified as areas in which the students needed additional support.

Sitlington, Neubert, Begun, Lombard, and Leconte (1996) provided suggestions for using interviews to obtain information for transition planning. Whenever possible, interviews should be conducted in person, and the environment should be arranged to make the interviewee as comfortable as possible. The purpose of the interview should be stated and the individual assured that there are no right or wrong responses. A specific list of questions should be asked and clarification given as needed. Respondents should have sufficient time to answer, and care should be taken not to lead or bias their answers. Finally, responses should be recorded either during or immediately after the interview to ensure that information has not been forgotten.

Questionnaires, Surveys, and Checklists

In many cases, individuals other than the teacher are in the best position to assess students' strengths and needs, identify available or potential supports, and describe future opportunities. Questionnaires, surveys, and checklists can provide information that is not easily observable, such as people's beliefs or a student's medical history. For example, family members can be asked to complete *home inventories,* which typically consist of questions addressing the student's home and neighborhood environment, household routines and expectations, present and future goals, and family members' preferences and personal values. The Home Inventory Form developed by Allen (1988) asks students and family members to identify students' likes, dislikes, concerns, strengths, needs, and involvement in community activities. In addition, questionnaires and checklists can provide valuable information about a student's performance from the perspective of others involved in employment and community environments (e.g., employers, co-workers, community members). For example, Storey and Garff (1999) asked a job coach to complete a survey to rate students' social interaction integration before and after a co-worker intervention.

Informal Assessment Procedures

Event Recording Datasheet

Student: **Emily Raptor**   Date: **March 25**

Location: **Lagner's Department Store**   Observer: **Ms. Roberts**

Activity: **Job training in the women's clothing section**

	Time	Greeted others	Asked for assistance	Provided assistance	Items folded correctly	Items folded incorrectly
	9:00–9:15	III	II	II	IIII II	I
	9:15–9:30	II	III	IIII	IIII	IIII
	9:30–9:45	—	II	I	IIII	—
	9:45–10:00	IIII	I	—	IIII IIII II	III
Total	1 hour	9	8	7	28	9

Comments: **Emily greeted only employees she knew well and very few customers. She increased the number of items she folded correctly by almost 10 over her last effort. She seems to really enjoy working around her friend Jane.**

Figure 5.1. Event recording datasheet for Emily Raptor. (From Hughes, C., & Carter, E.W. [2000]. The transition handbook: Strategies high school teachers use that work [p. 144]. Baltimore: Paul H. Brookes Publishing Co.; reprinted by permission.)

Interest Inventories

Research shows that students with severe disabilities often have little opportunity to make choices and decisions or express preferences (Wehmeyer & Metzler, 1995). Interest inventories can be used in conjunction with additional assessment procedures (e.g., direct observation or interviews) to identify current or potential areas of interest to guide transition planning (Clark, 1998). For example, a teacher may use an interest inventory to identify community activities in which a student would like to be involved, such as rock climbing or soccer. Next, the teacher would confirm the inventory results by actually observing the student engaging in those activities.

Although a number of commercial inventories exist, informal interest assessments can easily be developed by teachers. The items included on the interest assessment should relate directly to the purpose of the assessment (e.g., a career interest assessment should include items related to different occupations, working conditions, and potential job openings in the community). The format in which the assessment is given can be modified for students who have difficulty reading. For example, items can be presented verbally or visually, using pictures or videotapes to allow for the expression of a wide range of interest possibilities (Lohrmann-O'Rourke, Browder, & Brown, 2000).

Self-Assessments

Traditionally, students with disabilities have had little opportunity to actively participate in their own transition assessment process (Halpern, 1994). Self-assessment provides a means for students to evaluate their own performance and monitor their progress toward achieving a particular goal. Students can be taught to use checklists, rating scales, charts, graphs, pictures, or other means to assess and monitor their behavior. First, teachers should model appropriate use of the assessment procedure chosen, using corrective feedback as needed. Next, the student is taught to compare his or her performance with a set goal (Wehmeyer, Agran, & Hughes, 1998). For example, students have been taught to assess their performance in directing their own individualized education program (IEP) meetings (Martin, Marshall, Maxson, & Jerman, 1996). Students evaluate their behavior during their meetings on 11 previously instructed steps and their progress toward meeting their performance goals.

Social Support Assessment

As students approach adult life, the amount of social support they receive greatly influences the degree of success and satisfaction they experience. Social support may come from a variety of sources, such as friends of a student's brother or sister or someone who waits at the same bus stop to go to work. Social support assessment can assist practitioners in identifying the types of support available in an environment as well as additional support needed. By observing students and others as they interact throughout the day, interviewing important others, and surveying an environment, teachers can isolate sources of support that enhance students' performance and promote their social acceptance. For example, a social support assessment may reveal that employees in a publishing company have a walking club at noon and celebrate each others' birthdays during their breaks. Information gathered from the assessment can be used as the foundation for building an individual social support plan to allow a student to obtain existing support. Figure 5.2 shows an individual social support plan for Alfred Otawba, a young man who works at a bicycle shop and lives in an apartment with a roommate.

Ecological Inventories

Ecological inventories are typically used to assess relevant features of an environment or program. The information they yield is highly individualized to the specific demands of a particular situation and the relevant skills necessary for success in that environment (Rainforth & York-Barr, 1997). Ecological inventories can have a high degree of ecological validity because the information gathered from interviews, questionnaires, and informal observations is derived from the actual environment in which a student is or will be participating. One example of an ecological inventory is a job analysis survey, which provides relevant information about the environmental, social, and task characteristics of potential worksites (Benz, Yovanoff, & Doren, 1997). In addition, potential supports in the work environment that may increase a student's success on the job are identified. For example, features of worksites assessed by Renzaglia and Hutchins (1995) included type of job or position, job task requirements, task-related characteristics, environmental factors, and natural supports.

Step 5: Modify Procedures as Needed

Many students with severe disabilities have unique needs and forms of communicating. After selecting an appropriate informal assessment, practitioners may need to modify assessment procedures based on particular needs of the student and the characteristics of relevant environments. For example, Kraemer, Blacher, and Marshal (1997) modified an interview format in order to gather information from parents regarding the participation of high school students with severe disabilities in a variety of family and school activities. Findings showed that families wanted their adolescents to live and work independently, but few believed it would happen. Chadsey-Rusch, Linneman, and Rylance (1997) modified a survey to assess the beliefs of job coaches, employers, and students with intellectual disabilities regarding social integration outcomes and intervention procedures introduced in employment environments. Results revealed that although respondents agreed on the importance of some interventions and outcomes, they disagreed on others (e.g., task-related interactions).

Step 6: Conduct the Assessment

After selecting an informal assessment procedure and modifying it, if necessary, practitioners can begin conducting the assessment. For example, teachers and general education peers used a task analysis to assess the acquisition of leisure skills by four students with moderate disabilities (Collins, Hall, & Branson, 1997). Assessment took place after the assessment purpose was determined and target behaviors were verified by others. Findings indicated that none of the students with disabilities were initially able to perform all of the steps of the task analyses. Branham, Collins, Schuster, and Kleinert (1999) also used a task analysis to assess students' community skills (e.g., cashing a check, crossing the street, and mailing a let-

Individual Social Support Plan

Student's name: __Alfred Otawba__ Age: __20__ Date: __September 8__

	Support needs	Support strategy	Person or agency responsible	Outcome	Target date	Social needs
Vocational needs	• Improved job performance at the bike shop • Accepting criticism from supervisors	• Pair Alfred with another employee for continued job training. • Job coach and co-workers will model expected behavior.	• Vocational counselor will help co-worker adapt training. • Co-worker • Job coach • Adult service agency	• Alfred's job output will increase 20% • Alfred will say, "Thank you for the help," when given job feedback.	11/15 10/15	• Co-worker will record the number of bikes Alfred builds each week. • Direct observation and student interviews
Community needs	• Transportation training—needs way to get to the store, work, and various community activities	• Teacher/family will show how to use public transportation. • Friends will provide rides. • Co-workers will provide a ride to the worksite.	• Special education teacher • Parents • Peers • Co-workers	• Alfred will use public transportation to get to a desired location. • Alfred will contact and ride with a co-worker to his worksite.	11/15 10/15	• Log books and direct observation • Direct observation and communication with co-workers
Residential needs	• Planning meals that address Alfred's diet needs • Budgeting for monthly expenses	• Nurse trains roommate to help Alfred plan meals that meet his diet needs. • Teacher will provide classroom instruction. • Parents will help Alfred.	• Nurse • Alfred's roommate • General and special education teachers • Parents	• With the assistance of a roommate, Alfred will plan weekly meals that meet his diet needs. • Alfred will complete a monthly budget.	12/1 12/1	• Examine weekly menu of meals that Alfred plans • Direct observation and communication with parents
Social needs	• Involvement in an extracurricular activity • Increased class involvement during general education classes	• Peer joins Alfred when he attends an extracurricular activity of his choice. • Peer can model behavior • Teacher provides more chances for involvement.	• Peers • Peers • General education teacher • Educational assistant	• Alfred will participate in at least one extracurricular activity. • Alfred will increase his active involvement in class by 50%.	10/1 1/1	• Direct observation and conversation with peers • Direct observation and communication with teacher

Figure 5.2. Individual social support plan for Alfred Otawba. (From Hughes, C., & Carter, E.W. [2000]. The transition handbook: Strategies high school teachers use that work [p. 128]. Baltimore: Paul H. Brookes Publishing Co.; reprinted by permission.)

ter). Results showed that, after instruction, each student was able to complete each step of the task analyses with 100% accuracy.

In conducting informal assessments, practitioners must continually check that they are consistently focusing on the established purpose of the assessment and the chosen behaviors and environments of interest. In particular, if assessments are being conducted over time, without constant surveillance the original intent of the assessment may become obscured. In addition, practitioners must continue to obtain input from important others to ensure the validity of the focus of the assessment and the relevance of findings. Finally, when conducting assessments in everyday environments such as shopping malls, worksites, or recreation centers, it is critical that procedures used are nonintrusive and nonstigmatizing to students (Cooper & Browder, 1998).

Step 7: Use Assessment Findings to Identify Transition Goals and Objectives

Assessment is not an end in itself. Instead, the most important function of transition assessment is to gather information that will inform and guide instruction, planning, and the provision of supports (Smith et al., 1996). In addition, practitioners must communicate this information in ways that are understandable to other transition team members, including students and their families. Based on assessment findings, the team then develops transition goals and objectives to guide students' educational programs.

When identifying transition goals and objectives, practitioners should consider the information gathered on both the student and the current and future environments in which he or she participates or is expected to participate. Assessment information related to the student's interests, preferences, strengths, skills, and needs should be compared with information concerning the environmental demands and supports that the particular student will encounter (Sitlington et al., 1996). Areas in which student competence needs to be increased or supports developed or enhanced, such as increasing attendance at school or work, should be targeted as potential goals and objectives. For example, Collins et al. (1997) choose to address leisure skills as an instructional goal for four students with moderate disabilities who were unable to perform all of the steps of a leisure skills task analysis. In addition, when prioritizing transition goals and instructional objectives, team members—including students and their families—should work together, continually soliciting input from each other.

Step 8: Develop Curricular Plans to Achieve Goals

The final step in the process involves the development of curricular plans to achieve the goals that have been identified for a student. Practitioners must identify relevant educational experiences within which a student's goals and objectives can best be addressed. Knowlton (1998) emphasized that curricular plans must be personalized for each student, based on a complete assessment of his or her current strengths, needs, preferences, and projections of future performance, rather than on preestablished educational policies. Educational experiences should also occur in inclusive environments, including general education classes and activities, service learning experiences (Burns, Storey, & Certo, 1999), community-based instruction (Beck, Broers, Hogue, Shipstead, & Knowlton, 1994), and job training sites. For example, a student with a goal of identifying her career interests may enroll in several career preparation courses and sample multiple community jobs in order to identify her employment preferences. Finally, practitioners must continue to conduct ongoing informal assessment to determine if students are making progress toward their transition goals and if students and important others are satisfied with the educational program.

APPLICATION OF THE MODEL

To illustrate application of our proposed informal assessment model, consider again the story of Lucinda and Mr. Perez shared at the beginning of the chapter. Had Mr. Perez used an informal assessment process that followed the eight-step model proposed in this chapter to identify a potential job for his student, Lucinda, the outcomes likely would have been different. Let's revisit each step of model in practice.

Mr. Perez Learns How to Assess

Spring semester was fast approaching and Mr. Perez had to make a decision regarding Lucinda's first job placement. In the past, he had simply placed students at one of three worksites depending on their test scores. This year, however, he had just attended a workshop on conducting informal assessment using an eight-step model. He decided that he would try the model with Lucinda.

Step 1: Determine the Purpose of Assessment

Since her freshman year, Lucinda had talked about wanting to get a job with her friends. As a member of her transition team, Mr. Perez, Lucinda's teacher, was helping develop an individualized transition plan for Lucinda. A myriad of question swirled around his head. Which jobs would best match her strengths and interests? What tasks would she have to do, and who would help her? Would she get along well with her co-workers? Mr. Perez wanted to help Lucinda identify her career interests, employment strengths, and support needs. He determined that identifying Lucinda's employment interests and performance across several types of jobs would be the purpose of his assessment efforts.

Step 2: Identify Relevant Behaviors and Environments

Mr. Perez knew that as far as Lucinda was concerned, it was a job at Skyedale Mall or no job at all! So, he decided to conduct the assessments at actual businesses in the mall. After all, those were the jobs she was considering, and that is where she

Informal Assessment Procedures

would be expected to demonstrate good work performance. He decided to get input from Lucinda and her family in order to select three or four jobs that Lucinda could try out. Then, he would focus particular attention on assessing Lucinda's work performance in relation to the demands of each of those job environments.

Step 3: Verify Steps 1 and 2 Based on Input from Student and Important Others

Mr. Perez confirmed the assessment plan with Lucinda! A job at the mall would allow her to earn money *and* hang out with her friends—two of her favorite activities. She added that she was worried about how businesses would accommodate her wheelchair. Also, Lucinda emphasized that she *did not* want to be embarrassed in front of her friends during the assessments! Because Lucinda was approaching the end of high school, her parents wanted to make sure that only jobs with career possibilities were considered. Other members of the transition team agreed.

Step 4: Choose Appropriate Assessment Procedures

In order to identify the types of job sites in which Lucinda would find the most enjoyment and success, Mr. Perez would begin by *interviewing* and *surveying* Lucinda and her parents. Based on the information he obtained, Mr. Perez would conduct a *job analysis* of several of the jobs they identified. Finally, he would use *direct observation* by having Lucinda try out each job to determine how she would perform under the various environmental, social, and task demands of each job in relation to available supports. Because he wanted more than one perspective on Lucinda's performance, he decided that he would also *interview* employers and co-workers regarding Lucinda's performance.

Step 5: Modify Procedures as Needed

Mr. Perez developed an interview and survey form to address only the types of jobs available in the Skyedale Mall. Also, he decided to take Lucinda to the mall to directly observe her impressions of the different jobs available. Because of the extent of Lucinda's support needs, Mr. Perez decided to expand the *supports* sections of the job analysis to focus on co-worker, supervisor, and environmental supports.

Step 6: Conduct the Assessment

Lucinda and her family indicated that Heritage Books, Zazzy's clothing store, and Bradford's department store might be good matches for Lucinda's interests, strengths, and needs. Mr. Perez approached the businesses that Lucinda and her family had prioritized and arranged for Lucinda to work at each one as he gathered information related to the demands of and supports available in the job environment. As promised, he was especially careful to be very discreet while observing Lucinda, sometimes posing as a customer!

Step 7: Use Assessment Findings to Identify Transition Goals and Objectives

After observing Lucinda at each of the businesses, the assessment results were clear to everyone—Lucinda was hooked on Zazzy's and wanted to pursue a job there. Information from Lucinda's work performance evaluation also revealed that she had difficulty completing certain job tasks, working continuously for long periods of time, and following her schedule. After discussing the findings with Lucinda and the rest of her transition team, Mr. Perez decided to focus on these objectives with the goal of maintaining supported employment.

Step 8: Develop Curricular Plans to Achieve Goals

Mr. Perez worked with the school counselor to enroll Lucinda in the work-study program. Lucinda, along with a job coach, went to work at Zazzy's three afternoons a week. The goal was to decrease the presence of the job coach by helping Lucinda to become more independent on the job and to obtain existing support, such as her posted instructions to employees and her fellow workers. Mr. Perez continued to assess Lucinda's progress and her satisfaction with the job as well as that of her parents and her supervisor.

SUMMARY

Appropriate, comprehensive, and ongoing assessment is critical to effective planning and programming for the transition from high school to adult life. For students with severe disabilities, assessment must be individualized and related directly to the actual contexts in which these students participate. In this chapter, we have proposed a model for guiding teachers in selecting and conducting appropriate informal assessment procedures for the purpose of transition planning. The model is composed of eight steps that direct practitioners in implementing an informal assessment process and translating assessment findings into individualized goals and curricular plans. By using this model, practitioners may help ensure that the instruction and support that students receive are both effective and relevant. Ultimately, use of the model may help increase the likelihood that high school students will achieve valued life goals.

REFERENCES

Agran, M., & Morgan, R.L. (1991). Current transition assessment practices. *Research in Developmental Disabilities, 12,* 113–126.

Allen, W.T. (1988). *Read my lips: It's my choice.* . . . St. Paul, MN: Governor's Council on Developmental Disabilities, Department of Administration.

Beck, J., Broers, J., Hogue, E., Shipstead, J., & Knowlton, H.E. (1994). Strategies for functional community-based instruction and inclusion of children with mental retardation. *Teaching Exceptional Children, 26,* 44–48.

Benz, M.R., Lindstorm, L., & Yovanoff, P. (2000). Improving graduation and employment outcomes of students with disabilities: Predictive factors and student perspectives. *Exceptional Children, 66,* 509–529.

Benz, M.R., Yovanoff, P., & Doren, B. (1997). School-to-work components that predict post-school success for students with and without disabilities. *Exceptional Children, 63,* 151–165.

Branham, R.S., Collins, B.C., Schuster, J.W., & Kleinert, H. (1999). Teaching community skills to students with moderate disabilities: Comparing combined techniques of classroom simulation, videotape modeling, and community-based instruction. *Education and Training in Mental Retardation and Developmental Disabilities, 34,* 170–181.

Burns, M., Storey, K., & Certo, N.J. (1999). Effect of service learning on attitudes towards students with severe disabilities. *Education and Training in Mental Retardation and Developmental Disabilities, 34,* 58–65.

Campbell, P.C., Campbell, C.R., & Brady, M.P. (1998). Team environmental assessment mapping system: A method for selecting curriculum goals for students with disabilities. *Education and Training in Mental Retardation and Developmental Disabilities, 33,* 264–272.

Chadsey-Rusch, J., Linneman, D., & Rylance, B.J. (1997). Beliefs about social integration from the perspectives of persons with mental retardation, job coaches, and employers. *American Journal on Mental Retardation, 102,* 1–12.

Clark, G.M. (1998). *Assessment for transitions planning.* Austin, TX: PRO-ED.

Collins, B.C., Hall, M., & Branson, T.A. (1997). Teaching leisure skills to adolescents with moderate disabilities. *Exceptional Children, 63,* 499–512.

Cooper, K.J., & Browder, D.M. (1998). Enhancing choice and participation for adults with severe disabilities in community-based instruction. *Journal of The Association for Persons with Severe Handicaps, 23,* 252–260.

Farley, R.C., & Johnson, V.A. (1999). Enhancing the career exploration and job-seeking skills of secondary students with disabilities. *Career Development for Exceptional Individuals, 22,* 43–54.

Halpern, A.S. (1994). The transition of youth with disabilities to adult life: A position statement of the Division on Career Development and Transition, the Council for Exceptional Children. *Career Development for Exceptional Individuals, 17,* 115–124.

Hughes, C., Killian, D.J., & Fischer, G.M. (1996). Validation and assessment of conversational interaction intervention. *American Journal on Mental Retardation, 100,* 493–509.

Hughes, C., Rodi, M.S., Lorder, S.W., Pitkin, S.E., Derer, K.R., Hwang, B., & Cai, X. (1999). Social interactions of high school students with mental retardation and their general education peers. *American Journal on Mental Retardation, 104,* 533–544.

Individuals with Disabilities Education Act Amendments of 1997, PL 105-17, 20 U.S.C. §§ 1400 *et seq.*

Janney, R.E., Snell, M.E., Beers, M.K., & Raynes, M. (1995). Integrating students with moderate and severe disabilities into general education classes. *Exceptional Children, 61,* 425–439.

Knowlton, E. (1998). Considerations in the design of personalized curricular supports for students with developmental disabilities. *Education and Training in Mental Retardation and Developmental Disabilities, 33,* 95–107.

Kraemer, B.R., Blacher, J., & Marshal, M.P. (1997). Adolescents with severe disabilities: Family, school, and community integration. *Journal of The Association for Persons with Severe Handicaps, 22,* 224–234.

Lim, L.H.F., & Browder, D.M. (1994). Multicultural life skills assessment of individuals with severe disabilities. *Journal of The Association for Persons with Severe Disabilities, 19,* 130–138.

Lohrmann-O'Rourke, S., Browder, D.M., & Brown, F. (2000). Guidelines for conducting socially valid systematic preference assessments. *Journal of The Association for Persons with Severe Disabilities, 25,* 42–53.

Macfarlane, C.A. (1998). Assessment: The key to appropriate curriculum and instruction. In A. Hilton & R. Ringlaben (Eds.), *Best and promising practices in developmental disabilities* (pp. 35–60). Austin, TX: PRO-ED.

Mactavish, J.B., Mahon, M.J., & Lutfiyya, Z.M. (2000). "I can speak for myself": Involving individuals with intellectual disabilities as research participants. *Mental Retardation, 38,* 216–227.

Martin, J.E., Marshall, L.H., Maxson, L.L., Jerman, P.A. (1996). *Self-directed IEP.* Longmont, CO: Sopris West.

Newton, J.S., Ard, W.R., & Horner, R.H. (1993). Validating predicted activity preferences of individuals with severe disabilities. *Journal of Applied Behavior Analysis, 26,* 239–245.

Park, H., Gonsier-Gerdin, J., Hoffman, S., Whaley, S., & Yount, M. (1998). Applying the participatory action research model to the study of social inclusion at worksites. *Journal of The Association for Persons with Severe Handicaps, 23,* 189–202.

Parsons, M.B., Reid, D.H., & Green, C.W. (1998). Identifying work preferences prior to supported work for an individual with multiple severe disabilities including deaf-blindness. *Journal of The Association for Persons with Severe Handicaps, 23,* 329–333.

Phelps, L.A., & Hanley-Maxwell, C. (1997). School-to-work transitions for youth with disabilities: A review of outcomes and practices. *Review of Educational Research, 67,* 197–226.

Rainforth, B., & York-Barr, J., (1997). *Collaborative teams for students with severe disabilities: Integrating therapy and educational services* (2nd ed.). Baltimore: Paul H. Brookes Publishing Co.

Ramasamy, R., & Taylor, R.L. (1996). Transition assessment: A critical process for students with disabilities. *Diagnostique, 21,* 59–62.

Reid, D.H, Parsons, M.B., & Green, C.W. (1998). Identifying work preferences among individuals with severe multiple disabilities prior to beginning supported work. *Journal of Applied Behavior Analysis, 31,* 281–285.

Renzaglia, A., & Hutchins, M. (1995). Materials developed for *A model for longitudinal vocational programming for students with moderate and severe disabilities.* Grant funded by the U.S. Department of Education, Office of Special Education and Rehabilitation Services.

Rosenthal-Malek, A. (1998). Assessment for instruction of students with developmental disabilities. In A. Hilton & R. Ringlaben (Eds.), *Best and promising practices in developmental disabilities* (pp. 35–60). Austin, TX: PRO-ED.

Sacks, S.Z., Wolffe, K.E., & Tierney, D. (1998). Lifestyles of students with visual impairments: Preliminary studies of social networks. *Exceptional Children, 64,* 463–478.

Siegel-Causey, E., & Allinder, R.M. (1998). Using alternative assessment for students with severe disabilities: Alignment with best practices. *Education and Training in Mental Retardation and Developmental Disabilities, 33,* 168–178.

Sitlington, P.L. (1996). Transition assessment: Where have we been and where should we be going. *Career Development for Exceptional Individuals, 19,* 159–168.

Sitlington, P.L., Neubert, D.A., Begun, W., Lombard, R.C., & Leconte, P.J. (1996). *Assess for success: Handbook on transition assessment.* Reston, VA: Council for Exceptional Children.

Sitlington, P.L., Neubert, D.A., & Leconte, P.J. (1997). Transition assessment: The position of the division on career development and transition. *Career Development for Exceptional Individuals, 20,* 69–79.

Smith, F., Lombard, R., Neubert, D., Leconte, P., Rothenbacher, C., & Sittlington, P. (1996). The position statement of the Interdisciplinary Council on Vocational Evaluation and Assessment. *Career Development for Exceptional Individuals, 19,* 73–76.

Smith, R.M. (1997). Varied meanings and practice: Teachers' perspectives regarding high school inclusion. *Journal of The Association for Persons with Severe Handicaps, 22,* 235–244.

Storey, K., & Garff, J.T. (1999). The effect of coworker instruction on the integration of youth in transition in competitive employment. *Career Development for Exceptional Individuals, 22,* 69–84.

Thompson, J.R., Fulk, B.M., & Piercy, S.W. (2000). Do individualized transition plans match the postschool projections of students with learning disabilities and their parents? *Career Development for Exceptional Individuals, 23,* 3–26.

Thurlow, M., & Elliott, J. (1998). Student assessment and evaluation. In F.R. Rusch & J.G. Chadsey (Eds.), *Beyond high school: Transition from school to work* (pp. 265–296). Bemont, CA: Wadsworth.

Vallecorsa, A.L., deBettencourt, L.U., & Garriss, E. (1992). *Special education programs: A guide to evaluation.* Park, CA: Corwin Press.

Wehmeyer, M.L., Agran, M., & Hughes, C. (1998). *Teaching self-determination to students with disabilities: Basic skills for successful transition.* Baltimore: Paul H. Brookes Publishing Co.

Wehmeyer, M.L., & Metzler, C.A. (1995). How self-determined are people with mental retardation? The national consumer survey. *Mental Retardation, 33,* 111–119.

York, J., & Tundidor, M. (1995). Issues raised in the name of inclusion: Perspectives of educators, parents, and students. *Journal of The Association for Persons with Severe Handicaps, 20,* 31–44.

Ysseldyke, J., & Olsen, K. (1999). Putting alternate assessments into practice: What to measure and possible sources of data. *Exceptional Children, 65,* 175–185.

6

Measuring What's Important
Using Alternative Assessments

Colleen A. Thoma and Mary Held

A VISION FOR THE FUTURE

Daniel sat in his transition planning meeting listening to others talk about the coming year. He was a senior in high school and looked forward to officially being an adult. He could already picture what life would hold for him and would talk about it in rich detail with his teachers, his mother, and most of his friends. He wanted to work with cars; he even picked out a local quick oil change shop in his neighborhood as the best possibility. He wanted to have his own apartment. He could cook some meals and regularly spent time at home alone when his mother was working late or taking college classes. Daniel was well-known and liked in his neighborhood, and he wanted to keep the connections with people there who he knew and liked. He often would spend time talking with the volunteers at the local fire station. He planned to keep those connections.

In the meeting, he listened to the plans for his transition out of high school. For work-related goals, he heard them plan for a job at a local bagel store where he could clean up and make coffee. When he spoke up and said what he would really like to do, he was told that it was too dangerous. The conversation returned to the possibilities at the bagel store. For recreation, the team's goal for him included joining the local Young Men's Christian Association (YMCA), where he could exercise, something he liked to do at home. Daniel was told that he needed to do more things with others. The team decided that he would do best if he lived in an apartment with support; the residential agency supervisor said that she knew of an opening in an apartment building where they had other "clients" living. The apartments were in a "secure" building, and the majority of the people who lived there were older adults or people with significant disabilities. It was across town from where he lived with his mother, far from the people he knew and who knew him.

At graduation, the goals from Daniel's transition plan were met. He was moving into the apartment in the secure building. He had a job at the bagel store, and the manager was asking him to work additional hours at her other store, too. He went to the local YMCA twice per week with his teacher. He was planning for his graduation party. Daniel told his mother, his teacher, his job coach, and most of his friends that he was excited to be graduating because then he could quit his job and stop going to the YMCA because there would not "be all of those people on my back."

REEVALUATION OF TRADITIONAL ASSESSMENT

Daniel's story describes an assessment that led to less than optimal postschool outcomes and a quality of life that was not what Daniel wanted. Because the team viewed his performance through the lens of traditional assessment, they did not gather information that allowed them to capture the essence of Daniel. They were therefore unable to successfully support Daniel in constructing an accurate picture of his "strengths, needs, preferences, and interests" that would lead to an "enhanced quality of life." His story is certainly not an isolated incident. The problem with the status quo is that in spite of all our best intentions and efforts, so far students with disabilities are still leaving high school with their dreams unmet. They are without the jobs, supports, and social lives they want (Louis Harris and Associates, 2000; Thurlow & Elliott, 1998). Hopefully, this kind of scenario will disappear once transition decisions are made with concrete information about a student's specific strengths and needs.

Transition planning for students with disabilities should begin with a comprehensive assessment strategy. The requirements of the Individuals with Disabilities Education Act (IDEA) of 1990 (PL 101-476) state that individual transition goals be based "upon student interests and preferences, taking into account their strengths and needs" (34 CFR, Section 300.18). This mandate further requires that special educators, transition coordinators, parents, and other support providers use multiple strategies to ensure that they have clearly heard and understood student preferences. Beyond the legal requirements, best practices in special education in general also demand that goals and objectives be based on accurate assessment results that uncover student preferences and interests. "A well-planned and executed assessment that results in each team member having a well-balanced understanding of a student's performance is one of the most important contributions to generating critical objectives, effective instruction, and meaningful outcomes" (Gilles & Clark, 2001, p. 80).

This chapter focuses on some other ways of gathering accurate and important information for and with high school students. It will examine a growing trend in the area of assessment, that of using alternative assessments. Case examples from the research of the authors will be used to highlight the issues and provide a real-life foundation for the discussion. The first part of the chapter examines the status quo in transition assessment and planning with an emphasis on why alternatives to traditional standardized measures are needed. The second section describes the array of best practice alternative assessment strategies that can enhance the transition assessment process, with examples of how these strategies were used to support the transition assessment and planning process for Jackson.

The first question many special educators ask when told about alternative assessments is "Why do we need alternatives?" Menchetti and Piland pointed out that "traditional approaches to assessment may not be sufficiently comprehensive to measure all areas that students with more severe disabilities require for quality of life enhancement" (2001, p. 233). In developing wise transition plans for and with students, teachers are interested in performance, that is, how well a student performs within a specific curriculum or environment. They are also interested in determining a student's preferences and interests in a variety of transition planning areas: community living, employment, postsecondary education, and so forth. Lastly, they are trying to determine what supports a student needs to make these preferences and interests possible, or probable. As Sitlington, Neubert, and Leconte described, "Transition assessment is the ongoing process of collecting data on the individual's strengths, needs, preferences, and interests as they relate to the demands of current and future working, educational, living, and personal and social environments" (1997, p. 71).

This way of looking at assessment is different from what has been done in the past. Then, student performance was measured in a decontextualized way using a snapshot approach with standardized tests. The result was information that served the adults on the transition team rather than the student and had little to do with the student's "strengths, needs, preferences, and interests" or how the student could perform in the real world. It also produced students who were disengaged from the assessment process.

Prior to the transition planning meeting, professionals prepared by collecting assessment information for the student about his or her impairments or needs (Thoma, Rogan, & Baker, 2001). These assessments typically included standardized test results, interest inventory surveys, curriculum-based measurements, and teacher or other professional observations. The results of these assessments were shared with the team, along with information about student progress on the previous year's goals (including behavior plans), school records, and reports from medical or other related services personnel.

During the meetings, which were held once per year, adult team members used the information collected to make decisions about student annual goals, short-term objectives, and necessary formal supports. There was a particular focus on the level of support as well as linking students to adult service agencies. These meetings worked to fit students into a program instead of trying to understand the student's dream and building learning experiences and supports that would make the dream a reality. If the student was present, adults rarely varied their interaction styles, talking around the student or including him or her only minimally in the decision-making process. Meetings could be reconvened, but this typically happened only in response to crisis situations.

The written plan developed in this meeting was based on a deficit model: The goals within them focused on remediation of what students could not do. Outcomes were based on a continuum of adult services. Often the written goals and objectives had little connection to student interests, preferences, and dreams and were not tied to real-world standards and criteria. In addition, these decisions were often made based on school- and districtwide policies related to functional curricula, inclusion, community-based instruction, and/or transition "programming." Placement was based on standardized test scores. The evaluation of student progress was typically accomplished through the use of standardized or norm- and/or criterion-referenced measures. Little attention was paid to real-world performance tasks.

The use of alternative, authentic assessment procedures, particularly a portfolio, can provide an opportunity for students to be more involved in the processes of choosing transition goals and evaluating their progress toward the goals. These assessment procedures can also change the focus of transition planning from student deficits to student abilities by demonstrating student progress toward meeting goals, not just student progress on taking tests. Table 6.1 outlines distinctions between traditional transition assessment strategies and alternative assessment strategies.

CHARACTERISTICS OF ALTERNATIVE ASSESSMENTS

Alternative assessments are those processes and procedures that allow teachers to gather information about student progress using a multitude of methods and sources of information over time. They require that students construct a response rather than choose from two, four, or more response options (Mabry, 1999). This reliance on multiple processes and multiple sources of information lends itself well for use with students with various disabilities but particularly those with significant support needs who have a difficult time demonstrating what they know using conventional paper and pencil tests.

There are many definitions of alternative assessments and many types of alternative assessments. Some of these terms are used interchangeably. An examination of the vocational portion of the transition assessment plan for Jackson, a high school student, will highlight the major alternative assessment concepts. Jackson is an 18-year-old high school student with a love for cooking, being outdoors, fishing, hunting, and cute girls. His dream is to be a fisherman, although lately he is thinking seriously about becoming a cook. His teacher uses the Next S.T.E.P.: Student Transition and Educational Planning (Halpern et al., 1997) curriculum as a framework for her classroom. For the last 3 years, Jackson and his teacher have been using a transition portfolio that his teacher designed based on Next S.T.E.P. The purpose of the portfolio is to give Jackson and his teacher a systematic organized way to track the progress he makes toward achieving his goals and to provide a place to collect what is important to both of them.

Table 6.1. Comparison between current individualized education program (IEP) and individualized transition plan (ITP) process and an IEP and ITP process using alternative assessments

Current IEP and ITP process	Alternative IEP/ITP process
Information gathering Norm/criterion referenced Past school records Medical and related services reports Strengths/needs assessment based on observation Behavior plans/reports Possibly, parent surveys, student interviews These are the lowest priority and are often done in the meeting itself without preparation.	**Information gathering** Multiple measures Student involved in assessing own capacities Parent interview important piece of information Teacher observations Significant other input: friends, boyfriends or girlfriends, relatives, neighbors Activity folder contents (videotaped observations, demonstrations of mastery, performance tasks, projects)
Case conference process Focus on deficits/remediation Adults (professionals and at times, parents) make decisions for student Plan postschool supports Plan annual goals and objectives with individualized standards/criteria Focus on linking to adult service agencies Meet annually with not much preplanning or follow-up Could reconvene meetings; decision in hands of adults	**Case conference process** Student-led (to the extent possible) with support during and preparation prior to meeting Develop student decision-making skills Develop student self-advocacy skills Focus on student-identified goals and strengths Professionals support student decisions Plan for postschool outcomes Plan annual goals and objectives based on student's adult life goals and general education curriculum Identify supports student wants to achieve adult lifestyle Meet quarterly with ongoing support from committee members Decision to reconvene can come from student
Content of plan Curriculum is categorized: educational goals developed first; then rearranged into transition areas. Little connection between goals or between goals and student plans for adult lifestyle. Individualized goals and objectives Teacher plans instructional strategies, materials, and adaptations based on annual goals and objectives Curriculum will vary based on school's policies regarding inclusion, community-based instruction, perceived support needs of student, and school-to-career or transition "programs" Class placement is based upon standardized test scores	**Content of plan** Focus on transition-planning or adult lifestyle areas Individualized goals and objectives Student, with committee support, plans instructional strategies, materials, and adaptations based on annual goals and objectives and learning strengths and preferences Curriculum/class placement will vary based on student's desired adult goals

(continued)

Table 6.1. *(continued)*

Current IEP and ITP process	Alternative IEP/ITP process
Evaluation of progress Norm/criterion-referenced assessment and/or summative tests Multiple measures not necessarily authentic	**Evaluation of progress** Assessment features: multiple measures; authentic, performance-based assessments; personalized Students will keep activity folders/files that will be a collection of all work completed during year Contents of activity folder will be reviewed quarterly by team members and student Contents of portfolio will be chosen from contents of activity folder, with at least one entry for each transition planning area. Contents will be chosen to reflect progress over time, not just end result. Contents will be evaluated by experts in area/field for accountability purposes.

DEFINITIONS

There are many types and characteristics of alternative assessment strategies that can be used as part of a transition assessment process. This section will define these terms and strategies with examples of how they were used to guide Jackson's transition planning and assessment process.

Performance Assessment

Performance assessments are those assessments that "require students to generate rather than choose a response; [they] require students to actively accomplish complex and significant tasks while bringing to bear prior knowledge, recent learning, and relevant skills to solve problems" (Herman, Aschbacher, & Winters, 1992, p. 2). In Jackson's case, the tasks being assessed are the individualized education program (IEP) goals with benchmarks related to the work outcome of *becoming a cook* that he wrote with his teacher. Assessment was not separate from learning; rather, the two were integrally linked. His goals for this area were to

- Interview practicing cooks at area restaurants
- Tour the chef program at the vocational school
- Take a cooking class in school
- Work as a cook through the work-study program at the school

Authentic Assessment

Authentic assessments are those assessments that "require that students actively accomplish complex and significant tasks that are similar to tasks performed by adults in the real worlds of work, community living, recreation and leisure, and other aspects of everyday life" (Wiggins, 1993, p. 215). Prior to writing IEP goals and benchmarks and based on his interest in becoming a cook, Jackson and his teacher worked very hard to find out how people become cooks. What classes do they take in high school? Do they learn on the job, go to a vocational school, or attend college? Jackson's learning about his preferences, interests, and abilities came about by trying them out in inclusive classes at school and through opportunities in the community.

Formative and Summative Assessments

Formative assessments are those assessments that take place over time, measuring or recording student progress during that time. *Summative assessments* are those assessment procedures that measure student achievement at one point in time at the end of instruction or an instructional period of time (i.e., semester, quarter, or academic year). Each of Jackson's goals had benchmarks associated with it and evidence of the process (how he accomplished the goal), and the finished product was collected. For example, before each interview with a practicing cook, Jackson and a teaching assistant generated the questions he wanted to ask. During the interview, Jackson took notes, and the teaching assistant supported Jackson by writing down the responses. After each interview, the teacher went over this information with Jackson and asked him to write one paragraph about what he had learned (formative). After all of the interviews, Jackson was required to review all the paragraphs, synthesize the information using questions that the teacher generated, and give an oral report to the teacher about what he needed to do to become a practicing cook (summative).

Portfolios

Portfolios are "collections of information by and about a student to give a broad view of his or her achievement" (Mabry, 1999, p. 17). A portfolio can include samples of student work, narrative descriptions, résumés, grades, official records, student reflection or self-evaluation, responses from parents and/or bosses, and radio or photographic records. Portfolios can be artifacts or electronic records of such artifacts. Many schools are moving toward electronic portfolios that allow videotaped and/or audiotaped samples of student performances to be included.

In Jackson's portfolio, evidence of both process and product are included. In the front of the portfolio box is a laminated visual of Jackson's Planning Alternative Tomorrows with Hope (PATH; Pearpoint, O'Brien, & Forest, 1993). Next is a folder with sheets designed by the teacher so that Jackson can track the progress he is making toward meeting his goals. In the next folder, there is an abundance of *problem-solving sheets* that he can use if he runs into any difficulty while completing tasks. The portfolio is divided by the major transition planning areas identified in Next S.T.E.P. (personal life, education and training, living on my own, and jobs). Each major section is further subdivided by his IEP goals.

Demonstrations of Mastery

Demonstrations of mastery are typically formal, public performances of student competence and skill that provide an opportunity for a summative or final assessment. Demonstrations may also be formative, ongoing, informal, and embedded in curricula and everyday practices. Performances may be supported by tangible products, results of experiments, or solutions to practical problems. Jackson works as a cook at a fast-food restaurant near his school with the support of a teaching assistant. He makes hamburgers during the lunch hour. One of his goals is to increase the number of hamburgers that he can cook during the time he is there. Jackson has a form that he uses to record the number each day, and the teaching assistant helps him by counting as Jackson finishes making a hamburger. Once each grading period, his teacher comes by to watch him work and make suggestions for how he might improve.

Discourse Assessment

Discourse assessment provides students with an opportunity to tell others what they know. Typically by talking with an assessor, the student indicates what he or she has learned, offering evidence of critical thinking or problem-solving skills by producing narratives, arguments, explanations, original summaries, interpretations, analyses, or evaluations. The assessor listens and probes for evidence of achievement, such as responses that integrate relevant and important knowledge within a particular field and adapt and apply knowledge to novel problems or situations. Whenever Jackson and his teacher meet, they discuss how he is doing on meeting goals and benchmarks. As in the example at the beginning of this section, they discuss what he's learned and talk about any problems that have arisen.

Projects

Projects are question-oriented assignments that are specialized and often interdisciplinary. They are undertaken by a student or group of students. Project work results in personalized (and perhaps new) knowledge, idiosyncratic competencies, subtle skills, and professional-like motivation and habits. One of the projects that Jackson did was to research on the Internet to do a report about cooking as a career. A peer worked with him to develop a list of questions to be answered and to support his use of the Internet. As they discovered answers to questions, the peer took notes for Jackson. Jackson also found pictures that he liked featuring cooks and printed them out. He used the computer to write the report using report guidelines and standards developed by his teacher.

Profiles

Profiles are collections of ratings, descriptions, and summary judgments by teachers and sometimes by the student and others to give a broad view of his or her achievement. A profile typically includes a variety of contents, which may vary from checklists to certificates to narrative descriptions of what a student knows and can do. It may document academic achievement, nonacademic achievement, or both. Each student in Jackson's classroom has a personal profile that was developed by the teacher and student and contains very descriptive information. Its purpose is to give others a comprehensive but brief (one page) sense of the student and his or her level of performance as well as his or her preferences, interests, and support needs. The profile has three sections:

1. Who the student is—For Jackson, this part has his age, where and with whom he lives, his interests and preferences, what he likes and dislikes, and how he learns best.

2. What the student is good at—Information about strengths goes in this part. For example, in Jackson's profile it talks about cooking, fishing, hunting, being UNO champion, and charming girls.

3. What the student needs help with—This section contains information about areas that Jackson is working on improving and needs more intensive support around. For example, he is a student with a brain injury and needs help remembering and problem solving.

Performance Tasks

Performance tasks are

> Tasks, problems, or questions that require students to construct rather than select responses and may also require them to devise and revise strategies, organize data, identify patterns, formulate models and generalizations, evaluate partial and tentative solutions, and justify their answers. (Mabry, 1999, p. 17)

All of the learning or performance that Jackson is doing in the vocational area is based on questions that he and his teacher designed together. Because his goal is to explore the career of a cook, the major question is "What do I need to know and be able to do in order to become a cook?" All of the activities (interviewing, shadowing, cooking at the fast-food restaurant, and so forth) he does in order to answer this question are performance tasks. His teacher, who sees herself as a facilitator of learning, supports Jackson by helping him see connections, patterns, models, and so forth among tasks.

Simulation

Simulation is a task designed to incorporate problem-solving features similar to those found in practical or professional contexts. Simulations vary in the degree to which they mirror real-life situations and in the degree to which they offer structured or ill-defined tasks. Simulations may involve role-playing or computer delivery of tasks (Margolis, DeChaplain, & Klass, 1998). One simulation that Jackson and his classmates participated in was about job interviews. The teacher and students created a list of interview questions and standards of interview behavior. The students were paired up with peer tutors to practice asking and answering the questions. When each pair thought they were ready, a student from the videotape class at the high school made a videotape of the interview. After all the videotapes were completed, they were viewed by the class, and each pair was given peer and teacher feedback.

HOW DO WE MEASURE PROGRESS?

There are a number of different ways to "score" the work of students. Lewin and Shoemaker (1998) listed the following options: rubrics, checklists, assessment lists, and score cards. Regardless of the method used, Wiggins (1993) recommended that the scoring method provide clear standards and criteria to students so that they will know what is expected. In addition, Mabry recommended that there be flexibility in the criteria to give "credit for unique and unexpected aspects of performance" (1999, p. 35).

Rubrics

Rubrics are the most common scoring method for alternative, performance-based assessments. "A rubric is a set of scoring guidelines for evaluating student work" (Lewin & Shoemaker, 1998, p. 29). A rubric generally includes a scoring scale and a set of descriptors for each level of performance. They can be holistic or analytic (Lewin & Shoemaker, 1998). Holistic rubrics provide an opportunity for the assessor to look at student performance as a whole. Task-analytic rubrics divide a task into multiple traits and grades student performance in each of those trait areas. "Because rubrics describe levels of performance, they provide important information to teachers, parents, and others interested in what students know and can do. Rubrics also promote learning by offering clear performance targets to students for agreed-on standards" (Marzano, Pickering, & McTighe, 1993, p. 29). The contents of the rubrics are explained to students prior to their beginning a task so that they know exactly what is expected of them and what different levels of performance mean to them in terms of a score. The teacher in Jackson's class has written a holistic rubric for student portfolios and constructs rubrics for individual tasks that students are asked to do. She uses a grid that has the expected standards in one column and the levels of performance in the other.

Checklists

Checklists identify critical traits that must be present in the performance and provide opportunities for students to indicate the presence of the traits by checking them off as completed or not completed (Lewin & Shoemaker, 1998). This is an all or nothing assessment; it does not provide feedback about how well a task or trait was done, just whether it was done or not. Jackson's portfolio contains a folder that lists all of his goals and benchmarks. There is a checklist that he uses to mark the ones that he has finished so that he and his teacher know what he is working on.

Assessment Lists

Assessment lists, like checklists, indicate to students what essential traits of excellence must be present in the performance, but they go further (Lewin & Shoemaker, 1998). Assessment lists also provide a weighted scoring value for each trait. The teacher determines the relative importance of the traits by assigning a point value. Assessment lists provide students with an opportunity for self-assessment in a designated column, before receiving the teacher's evaluation of points earned in another column.

Jackson's portfolio contains information about his self-assessment of his behavior in the classroom. There are some things that he is working on that are less critical than others and, therefore, are weighted less than the others. For instance, Jackson wants to limit the amount of his singing in public, which is not a significant or priority goal; however, his goal to stop hitting others when he is upset and instead talk through his frustrations is a priority goal and therefore carries three times the weight of the first goal. He rewards himself with a walk outside when he hits 25 points, which takes less time when he catches himself meeting his priority goals.

Score Cards

Score cards contain analytical traits and a scoring scale (Lewin & Shoemaker, 1998). In addition, they add a point system that provides an overall score. This overall score can then be converted into a percentage or letter grade. Jackson's science teacher uses a scorecard to individualize Jackson's grade in the class. Grades consist of his participation in experiments, grades on quizzes, and his behavior as described in the assessment list. An *A* for the class must include full participation in the class, limitation of disruptive behavior, and performance on quizzes developed for him.

Student Self-Evaluation

Student self-evaluation received serious consideration as a valid means of assessment during the 1990s (Marzano et al., 1993). Particularly when assessment is part of a comprehensive transition planning process that encourages student self-determination, student self-evaluation provides an opportunity for students to participate in transition assessment and learn more about their own abilities. Journals are one self-assessment tool that have been used extensively, particularly in the area of literacy development (Atwell, 1987; Calkins, 1986; Macrorie, 1984). This strategy consists of an assessor providing a specific probe or question to students on their reading. Students write their answers to this probe in their journals, and the teacher reads them to check for specific standards (i.e., content knowledge, information processing, collaboration/cooperation, and so forth).

At the end of each task, Jackson is required to reflect on his learning and to complete a self-evaluation form that his teacher developed. The form asks students to summarize the completed activity; to say what they liked about the task, what they didn't like about it, what they did well, and what they needed help with; and to list any questions they have. They then circle the number on a scale of 1–5 (5 being the highest) to indicate how well they think they did on the task.

Other Evaluation and Feedback

Other evaluation or feedback to students is another unique feature of performance assessments. Although most other types of assessment provide information about student learning at a given point of time, performance assessments can provide information about student learning across time. In fact, the assessment process itself should be considered to be an important learning exercise. To do that, teachers provide ongoing feedback to students throughout the assessment process or during specific points throughout the process. Wiggins (1993) reported that good feedback is descriptive; it tells a student if he or she is "off-track (or on-track) without labeling or judging his [or her] efforts" (p. 188). Effective feedback, therefore, should provide 1) concrete, descriptive information about the expected performance; 2) exemplary standards for performance; 3) feedback about how a student is doing compared with the exemplar or expected performance; and 4) information about what a student can do to improve his or her performance (Gilbert, 1978). Although much of this feedback can be verbal, the "use of exemplars, rubrics, and performance troubleshooting guides or checklists used by individual students or in peer review, can go a long way toward providing good feedback" (Wiggins, 1993, p. 197).

After each performance task, Jackson gets feedback from his teachers and may also receive feedback from peers, supervisors, and co-workers. The teacher has designed a form that facilitates periodic feedback from others. Jackson meets daily with his teacher for support and feedback and to modify goals and benchmarks. At report card time (quarterly), meetings also serve the purpose of evaluating Jackson's overall progress toward his goals.

HOW CAN ALTERNATIVE ASSESSMENTS BE INFUSED INTO TRANSITION ASSESSMENT AND PLANNING?

The key to using alternative assessments successfully mirrors the key to all assessment: It is imperative that one begins by identifying what information is needed to assist the decision-making process. Wiggins and McTighe (1998) recommended using a backward design process. Step 1 is to identify the desired results or outcomes. For Daniel, the desired results or outcomes included working at an oil change shop, having his own apartment, and remaining in his neighborhood so that he could keep connections to his friends and social events.

Step 2 involves determining acceptable evidence. How will the planning team know if Daniel is able to accomplish these goals, and when will they know if he has achieved them? To identify this, transition team members need to share information that they already know about Daniel and allow him to share information he knows about himself. With all the types of assessment instruments and strategies available, it is easy to be overwhelmed. In Daniel's example, his transition planning team needed information to evaluate whether he could accomplish these goals. They had some information about his ability to fix things and his ability to cook some simple meals (from reports from his mother and neighbors). They needed to know whether he could work safely in an oil change shop and whether he could live on his own safely.

The first part of Step 2 is to identify tasks that would provide the team with the relevant information. Information gathered at an oil change shop and at home would provide the team with key information about whether Daniel could do these things now, as well as target areas for learning if he could not. Portfolios, especially electronic portfolios, could gather the information necessary over time that would answer these questions.

The second part of Step 2 is to determine the consequences of these assessment strategies. In Daniel's case, safety was an important consideration for work at the oil change shop. Team members would not allow him to work there without first determining whether these concerns were valid. Likewise, they would not let him live alone for a period of time without any supervision to see if he could do it. Instead, they would build up time spent alone in manageable increments as an alternative to "all or nothing" or "sink or swim" approaches.

Step 3 is to use the results of the assessment(s) to plan learning experiences. If Daniel was not able to work successfully at the oil change shop, the problems he had (his strengths and needs) would be evaluated to see what he needed to learn, and the best ways to teach this information. If the team and Daniel decided that working in an oil change shop was not something that would be appropriate for him, they would begin to help him learn about other alternatives based on what was learned from the assessment.

Table 6.2 outlines the different alternative assessment strategies and how they could have been used for Daniel. Obviously, it takes more than the use of alternative assessment approaches to ensure that wise transition plans are developed for students. Those who use these alternative approaches with students must adhere to the basic underlying values that ensure wise transition assessment and planning. For instance, alternative assessment strategies should not be used to limit student preferences and interests. They should not be used to limit the involvement of family members and to track students with disabilities into sheltered workshops, enclaves, and group homes.

The promise of alternative assessment strategies used in transition planning should be to respect the rights of students and parents to make choices for a quality of life. These strategies are essential for assuring a collaborative planning process in the best definition of the word and opening opportunities rather than limiting them unnecessarily. In sum, they need to support wise transition assessment and planning.

Table 6.2. Alternative assessment strategies that work

Strategy	Definition	Example
Portfolios	Collections of formal and informal information about student achievement containing samples of student work in one or more areas. All of the other types of assessment strategies could be included in a portfolio.	Daniel's completed portfolio was used to demonstrate his ability to meet his dreams for a job in the community, living in his own apartment, and being relatively independent in recreation and leisure activities. The works that he collected were chosen to best demonstrate his independence, productivity, and potential.
Demonstrations of mastery	Formal, more or less public performances of student competence or skill that provide opportunities for culminating assessments. These may be tangible products, experimental conclusions, or solutions to practical problems.	Daniel's ability to change oil in a car was assessed by the owner of a local automotive repair shop at the end of his on-the-job training program.
Performance tasks	Tasks, problems, or questions that require students to construct rather than select their own responses	Daniel's long-term dream includes living in his own apartment with minimal supports. The local agency that provides such support requires that adults first live in group homes that provide 24-hour coverage and demonstrate mastery of specific goals. Instead, Daniel's performance in those areas (responding to emergencies, cooking simple meals, and handling finances) was part of his annual assessment process.
Profiles	Ratings, descriptions, and summary judgments produced by teachers, students, parents, and others to give a broad view of student achievement	Daniel's profile focused on all areas of his adult life: his ability to work with cars, live in the community, and take the bus to and from work; his hobbies and recreation interests; and his relationships with others.
Projects	Original, often specialized inquiries devised and undertaken by a student or group of students	Projects for Daniel focused on his desire to live in his own apartment. His project involved collecting the information necessary to determine how this could become a reality for him. His research involved examining the social climate of various apartment complexes; the costs associated with living there (rent, membership fees, utilities); the amenities available; and the proximity to work, recreation, shopping, family, and friends. He also learned how to examine an apartment for problems (insect infestation, rusty plumbing, and structural problems).
Assessment of discourse	An evaluation of what students say. Through language, students indicate their learning by offering evidence of critical thinking or problem solving.	Daniel had a difficult time expressing himself in writing but had no problem telling others what he knew. Instead of taking a written history examination at the end of the semester, he verbally answered a series of questions supplied by his teacher and other students.

REFERENCES

Atwell, N.C. (1987). *In the middle.* Wesport, CT: Heinemann.

Calkins, L.M. (1986). *The art of teaching writing.* Wesport, CT: Heinemann.

Gilbert, T.F. (1978). *Human competence.* New York: McGraw-Hill.

Gilles, D., & Clark, D. (2001). Collaborative teaming in the assessment process. In S. Alper, D.L. Ryndak, & C.N. Schloss (Eds.), *Alternative assessment of students with disabilities in inclusive settings* (pp. 75–87). Needham Heights, MA: Allyn & Bacon.

Halpern, A., Herr, C.M., Wolf, N., Doren, B., Johnson, M., & Lawson, J. (1997). *Next S.T.E.P.: Student transition and educational planning.* Austin, TX: PRO-ED.

Herman, J.L., Aschbacher, P.R., & Winters, L. (1992). *A practical guide to alternative assessment.* Alexandria, VA: Association for Supervision and Curriculum Development.

Individuals with Disabilities Education Act (IDEA) of 1990, PL 101-476, 20 U.S.C. §§ 1400 et seq.

Lewin, L., & Shoemaker, B.J. (1998). *Great performances: Creating classroom-based assessment tasks.* Alexandria, VA: Association for Supervision and Curriculum Development.

Louis Harris and Associates. (2000). *The National Organization on Disability/Harris survey program on participation and attitudes: Survey of Americans with disabilities.* New York: Author.

Mabry, L. (1999). *Portfolios plus: A critical guide to alternative assessment.* Thousand Oaks, CA: Corwin Press.

Macrorie, K. (1984). *Writing to be read.* St. Portsmouth, NH: Boynton/Cook.

Margolis, M.J., DeChamplain, A.F., & Klass, D.J. (1998, April). *Comparing alternative procedures for scoring a performance assessment of physicians' clinical skills.* Paper presented at the annual meeting of the National Council on Measurement in Education, San Diego.

Marzano, R.J., Pickering, D., & McTighe, J. (1993). *Assessing student outcomes: Performance assessment using the dimension of learning model.* Alexandria, VA: Association for Supervision and Curriculum Development.

Menchetti, B.M., & Piland, V.C. (2001). Transition assessment and evaluation: Current methods and emerging alternatives. In S. Alper, D.L. Ryndak, & C.N. Schloss (Eds.), *Alternative assessment of students with disabilities in inclusive settings* (pp. 220–255). Needham Heights, MA: Allyn & Bacon.

Pearpoint, J., O'Brien, J., & Forest, M. (1993). *PATH: A workbook for planning positive possible futures.* Toronto: Inclusion Press.

Sitlington, P.L., Neubert, D.A., & Leconte, P.J. (1997). Transition assessment: The position of the Division on Career Development and Transition. *Career Development for Exceptional Individuals, 20*(1), 69–79.

Thoma, C.A., Rogan, P., & Baker, S. (2001). Student involvement in transition planning: Unheard voices. *Education and Training in Mental Retardation and Developmental Disabilities, 36*(1), 16–29.

Thurlow, M., & Elliott, J. (1998). Student assessment and evaluation. In F.R. Rusch & J.G. Chadsey (Eds.), *Beyond high school: Transition from school to work* (pp. 265–296). Belmont, CA: Wadsworth.

Wiggins, G. (1993). *Assessing student performance: Exploring the purpose and limits of testing.* San Francisco: Jossey-Bass.

Wiggins, G., & McTighe, J. (1998). *Understanding by design.* Alexandria, VA: Association for Supervision and Curriculum Development.

7

Assessing Individual Needs for Assistive Technology

Gerald Craddock and Marcia J. Scherer

WAITING FOR TECHNOLOGY

"For me it is very frustrating that it is now February, and I still haven't received my new assistive technology. I think that it is very unfair that students are made to wait until halfway through the academic year before they receive their equipment. I have been fortunate that my high school has allowed me to hang on to the computer I used to have, but other students who may be first-time users are not so lucky. Only this week, I talked to other students who could not cope with their college coursework without the necessary accommodations. We need to get our assistive technology before our academic year begins so that we can get it up and running. Maybe they should have started all this earlier . . ."

This passage was written by a student in his first year at University College Dublin. Sean received a personal computer while still in high school but was limited in using the keyboard in the traditional manner. Because he had significant physical disabilities, he was apprehensive about his ability to complete all the work expected at the postsecondary level. After going through an assistive technology (AT) assessment and having an opportunity to try out different types of equipment, Sean realized how much easier it would be to keep up with assignments by using AT. He received a mini-keyboard to accommodate his limited range of motion and a track-ball to use as a mouse. Sean was also provided the use of a scanner to cut down on the amount of physical effort required to hold books and turn pages. It was also helpful to listen to text instead of reading it all. He even got to try out the Dragon Naturally Speaking system; imagine speaking to the computer and having it type the right words. How he wished he had been introduced to all of this earlier!

IMPORTANCE OF ASSISTIVE TECHNOLOGY

Providing students with appropriate AT is challenging at best. When considering AT during high school years, extra attention must be paid to the potential use of AT as the student moves into other environments, including postsecondary education. This chapter focuses on the individual's role in obtaining appropriate AT and how wise practices can guide strategic decision making through transition and beyond.

Data from the U.S. Department of Education show that approximately 95% of students with disabilities are served in general education schools. Because students of all abilities are learning together in increasing numbers in public schools, the use of technology as an instructional, learning, and supplementary aid is changing the way teachers teach and children learn. For many students with disabilities, educational and assistive technology use is not a choice. AT is an essential means of keeping them active participants in their classrooms, assisting them to complete tasks that they cannot accomplish alone and enabling them to achieve the same instructional objectives as their peers without disabilities (Flemming & Flemming, 1995).

The importance of AT in the lives of people with disabilities was emphasized by Congress with the inclusion of AT in the Americans with Disabilities Act (ADA) of 1990 (PL 101-336); the Assistive Technology Act of 1998 (PL 105-394); the Individuals with Disabilities Education Act (IDEA) of 1990 (PL 101-476); and the Rehabilitation Act of 1973 (PL 93-112). IDEA further supports the use of AT by students with disabilities by stating that schools must provide AT for students at no cost to their parents if the student's individualized education program (IEP) team determines a need for the technology. Within the reauthorized IDEA Amendments of 1997 (PL 105-17), a new section focuses on the development of a student's IEP and the mandated consideration of AT devices and services. Identifying the supplementary supports and services needed to help students learn in general education classrooms using the general curriculum is also emphasized.

In spite of federal mandates for comprehensive, consumer-responsive AT and technology-related services, obtaining such devices and services often remains challenging for both the individual user and the school system. Today's educator is expected to be knowledgeable about a variety of technologies although he or she often has little opportunity and time to develop detailed expertise. There may be many hours of engineering and product testing for each AT device as well as manufacturers who staunchly stand by their products, but when matching a student with AT, educators are often very much alone. In addition, educators often feel responsible for achieving a good match between student and technology and for training the student with disabilities in its proper use. But the educator doesn't need to feel alone; in fact, the best partner is the student who is being matched with the technology.

Assessment components should be incorporated into AT evaluation procedures. Doing so will ensure that contextual factors and student learning preferences are addressed before AT is chosen. Information gathered should look at the comfort level and training of the users; the activity level; the time needed to customize or modify the device; and the identification of persons responsible for the integration, setup, and use of the AT in all of the environments that the technology will be used. Realistic expectations for AT outcomes by the family and professionals in the classroom, community, and home will affect the successful use of AT. As for the user, factors such as motivation to use the device, self-discipline to become more efficient with it, or the ability to cope with using a device that peers do not use will affect the successful integration of AT into the user's life.

REDUCING ASSISTIVE TECHNOLOGY NONUSE

Students' reactions to their ATs are individual and complex. Although ATs are designed to enhance learning, community participation, and independence, improved functioning by itself will not ensure AT use (Phillips & Zhao, 1993; Scherer, 1992, 2000; Scherer & McKee, 1990). Depending on the type of AT, nonuse (also called abandonment) can be as low as 8% or as high as 75%; on the average, one third of more optional ATs are abandoned, most within the first 3 months (Scherer & Galvin, 1994). The most frequently cited reasons for this were that the device was no longer needed and that the user did not have a say in which device was chosen.

One of the earliest studies to address the abandonment of recommended AT was conducted from 1975 to 1978. The Children's Hospital at Stanford (1980) conducted a follow-up study of the use of mobility aids over a 3-year period and found that 50% of the devices were being used an average of 9 hours per day. Twenty-two percent of the devices were no longer used. Sixty-nine percent of the study population was younger than 18 years old, and the primary reason for nonuse was that the device had been "outgrown."

Data from a study of AT abandonment among a sample of 227 American adults with a variety of disabilities yielded an overall device abandonment rate of 29.3% (Phillips & Zhao, 1993). Most abandoned devices were mobility aids, and most were abandoned either during the first year or after 5 years. The strongest factor influencing abandonment was a change in the needs or priorities of the user (either through improvement or decline in the person's functioning and medical condition, or other functional changes brought about by personal activities such as returning to work). Other strong influences on abandonment were how well the device performed; whether the user had a say in device selection; and whether the device met the user's expectations for effectiveness, reliability, durability, comfort, and ease of use.

A research study of adults with a variety of disabilities (Cushman & Scherer, 1996) sought to examine more closely the relationship between abandonment and functional improvement. One hundred twenty-eight devices were recommended to the 47 people in the study, an average of 2.7 per person. At the 3-month follow-up, 42 devices were no longer used, creating an overall nonuse rate of 33%. This rate of nonuse is consistent with studies cited previously.

The abandonment of grooming aids, manual wheelchairs, quad canes, and walkers was indeed tied to greater functioning in self-care and locomotion. Furthermore, a greater percentage of individuals who stated they no longer needed a recommended device actually showed functional improvement (versus those who continued using the device), but so did a large percentage of people who abandoned a device for other reasons. Other results indicated that users have positive expectations of devices and that if actual performance falls short of expectations, the response may be to stop using the device.

Together these results suggest that although functional improvement may lead to nonuse of recommended devices in many cases, other reasons for nonuse exist—especially when the person can get by without using the AT. If a student stops using his or her AT, ongoing evaluation and support should continue. Similarly, if an individual does not know how to use the device, possible modifications should be addressed in environments as close to "real use" situations as possible. In this way, an appropriate early intervention could be implemented in cases in which nonuse (for reasons other than functional improvement) is detected. This would help to identify individual training needs as well.

MATCHING PERSON AND TECHNOLOGY (MPT) MODEL

Successful AT use requires adapting the AT to the person's capabilities and temperament, not the other way around. It is also important to adapt the user, family, peers, co-workers, and others to the realities and situations of AT use. One useful method to organize the factors that influence a person's tendency to use an optional AT is the Matching Person and Technology (MPT) model (Scherer, 1998), which addresses three important components:

1. Characteristics of the environment and psychosocial setting in which the AT is used (Milieu)
2. Pertinent features of the individual's personality and temperament (Person)
3. Characteristics of the AT itself (Technology)

The United States and other countries need a valid assessment process that provides relevant and useful information for choosing appropriate AT devices. The MPT process has been effective in addressing and organizing the many influences that affect the use of AT, and this assessment tool is one that gathers information from a variety of sources through a set of instruments. It has been validated for use by people with disabilities ages 15 and older and has resulted in a high satisfaction of the selection of "useable" technology. It produces options that match not only the individual's strengths and needs but also consider his or her preferences and temperament. This information is then balanced with the characteristics of the environment that the technology will be used in (activity level, caregivers' and professionals' technology comfort level, and so forth) along with the characteristics of the technology itself. As an applied and research tool, it identifies barriers to AT use for a particular individual.

The MPT model is particularly useful as part of the transition process because all environments in which the AT is used, or might be used, must be considered. Applications of AT in postsecondary education, employment, and community activities must be assessed early on to identify necessary upgrades, modifications, or additional equipment that may be used in the future.

There are two companion forms in the present MPT instruments. Consumer and professional forms are designed to be used as a set so that 1) consumer input drives the MPT process, 2) professional and consumer perspectives can be compared, and 3) all relevant influences on technology use are considered. Based on the results of measurement standards, the MPT instruments have reasonable interrater reliability and validity (e.g., Crewe & Dijkers, 1995).

The MPT model consists of checklist-type assessment instruments to record the user's goals and preferences, views of the benefits to be gained from a technology, and changes in self-perceived outcome achievement over time. Each of the three components is first described in general terms; then, consideration for assessing these influences in transition settings are offered.

Identify the Environment

The environment(s) in which a person uses AT will either support or deter its use. Relevant features include the degree of social and economic support for technology use as well as the existence of physically accessible community features. In addition, factors such as environmental accommodations, available resources (e.g., special funding for specific equipment, availability of personal assistance), and special opportunities (e.g., access to high technology centers in postsecondary education) are important influences on AT use.

The availability of training for use of the equipment is crucial. Often, the device that worked so well in the rehabilitation facility does not work in the home or the classroom. The failure of ATs to fit well with the person's environment is a major reason for technology being abandoned. Another common reason for abandonment is that AT use was forced on the individual, and the AT immediately became a focal point for resentment.

The perspectives and expectations of others in the environment can be influential, especially if the technology inconveniences others. In this fast-paced world, it is often easier (and less emotionally painful) for family members to just jump in and do things for the person than to patiently step aside and watch the individual struggle to accomplish a task independently. Therefore, other people in the environment can nullify the individual's need for AT.

Assessing Milieu Influences

Trials of equipment in natural environments that involve everyone affected by the AT have proven to be cost effective long term because obstacles to optimal technology use can be identified before "bad habits" form. If, for example, a student is using alternate computer access in a computer lab in high school, he or she should try the same equipment in the high technology center of the community college. The environment may be very different, including the level of instructor and peer support, noise level, lighting considerations, and level of activity. Videotaping the use of equipment in different environments by a variety of students may help on both ends: for the student planning to attend postsecondary classes who can see what to expect in a new setting and for the professionals at both the sending and receiving institutions to identify solutions to potential obstacles.

Know the Person

When a person in the process of being matched with an AT is involved in selecting the equipment and encouraged to exercise choice regarding the equipment's features, the likelihood of the most appropriate AT being identified is improved. Many students and parents may see only limited alternatives for themselves because they have not been exposed to sufficient options to make informed choices and express appropriate preferences. The reaction by an individual who was born with a disability may differ significantly from that of someone who acquired a disability. Individuals who have not yet come to terms with their disabilities may not be able to exercise good judgment regarding AT selection. In addition, depression may mask capabilities and capacities that would erase the need for a technology. Introducing ATs too early may prevent the user from acquiring capacities and coping skills that take time to develop. As a result, the person may feel confused and frightened. Individuals who have a recent and severe disability due to trauma need to first be helped to understand their changed circumstances.

Assessing Characteristics and Preferences of the Person

Before a technology will be optimally used, a person must both need and want it. If an AT enhances the individual's self-esteem, self-efficacy, and overall quality of life, it will be used. Proper timing is of the essence. So is privacy. It is best to ask students about preferences, needs, and capabilities when their significant others and peers are not present. Significant others want to be helpful and should be involved, but it may be best to give them opportunities to express their preferences at another time. Sometimes, though, peers and family members are the best advocates, as Buswell and Sax describe in Chapter 4. In either case, the focus must remain on the student who will use the AT. If a student loves being the center of attention and demonstrates interest in and comfort with technology in general, then the likelihood of the AT being integrated increases. Some students do not want to stand out as being different from their peers. AT in this case must be chosen very carefully to include as few "bells and whistles" as possible.

Find the Best Technology

An AT device is abandoned when it is perceived as not being worth the effort required to set it up and operate it, is never there when needed, and is costly or inconvenient to maintain. Selecting the most appropriate technology with all the right features is a complex process. AT must have enough features to be useful and expandable but not so many that the user becomes overwhelmed. Overload is a concern when an individual already uses or is being matched with more than one technology. Multiple technology use can bring overload of many types—physical weakness, mental or emotional strain, and unwillingness to tolerate technical assistance.

For the most part and for a variety of reasons, people with disabilities have been socialized to minimize their disabilities. Again, equipment that makes an individual stand out in a crowd and eclipses the person using it has a high likelihood of being abandoned. Abandonment is also a probable outcome if the individual feels ostracized when using the technology and can get by without it.

Assessing Features of and Comparing Technologies

It has become increasingly difficult to keep up to date with new AT and improvements to existing ones. For this reason, the Technology Related Assistance for Individuals with Disabilities Act of 1988 (PL 100-407; reauthorized as the Assistive Technology Act of 1998, PL 105-394) was passed to help establish state AT centers. A major responsibility of these centers is to provide information about technologies and help individuals to obtain them. Equipment loan and trial programs, user and peer networks, and equipment funding assistance exist in many states. To find out the lead agency in a given state, contact RESNA Technical Assistance Project, 1700 North Moore Street, Suite 1540, Arlington, VA 22209-1903; (703) 524-6686; TTY: (703) 524-6639; http://www.resna.org.

EVALUATING AND DOCUMENTING
THE NEED FOR AND OUTCOMES OF ASSISTIVE TECHNOLOGY USE

Every match of person and technology requires careful consideration. Although some technologies are meant to be used for only a short time, premature AT abandonment is costly both in terms of dollars and outcome achievement regardless of whether the abandoned equipment is low technology (i.e., simple, using basic materials) or high technology (i.e., complex, electronic equipment). Equipment also becomes wasteful when it does not enhance the person's educational experience or performance—even if it is used. Professionals working with AT need to demonstrate that what AT does makes a difference and to assess and document outcomes of AT use.

When evaluating an individual for an assistive device, evaluation forms should be available that will guide professionals in considering those factors influencing an individual's predisposition to the use of an AT and to document that such consideration was done (e.g., Craddock, 2000). The MPT model is useful in documenting consumer goals and preferences, views of the benefits to be gained from a technology, and changes in self-perceived functioning and outcome achievement over time. It also flags potential mismatches between person and technology in the hopes that early identification of mismatches will:

1. Reduce technology nonuse or inappropriate use
2. Identify needed technology modifications
3. Eliminate frustration that occurs with a poor match of person and technology

Systematically implementing such a theory, or practice, requires a planned process of service delivery. An example of where this has been accomplished very effectively comes from the Republic of Ireland, where a 1-year demonstration project was conducted to develop a model of good practice in identifying the AT and training needs of students through the provision of a formal Statement of Assistive Technology Need prior to students who transition from second-level education (high school) to third-level education (college), employment, or vocational training.

A MODEL FOR THE FUTURE: THE IRISH STATEMENT PROJECT

Grant funds from the European Union's Horizon Programme allowed Client Technical Services (CTS) and the Central Remedial Clinic (CRC) to develop a model for the identification of AT and training needs of students transitioning from high school to college, vocational training, or work. The name of this project was Systematic Template for Assessing Technology Enabling Mainstream Education— National Trial (STATEMENT). The total number of students who applied to the project was 86, and the breakdown by disability type is shown in Table 7.1.

In Ireland, as elsewhere in Europe, the United States, and other countries, the evaluation of the needs of people with disabilities has traditionally been undertaken within the parameters of a medical model of disability (Craddock & Murphy, 1998). People with disabilities, however, "are challenging people to give up the idea that disability is a medical problem requiring 'treatment,' but to understand instead that disability is a problem of exclusion from ordinary life" (Central Remedial Clinic, 2000, p. 2). The need to establish evaluation systems informed by and consistent with the social model of disability (which focuses on physical, architectural, and attitudinal barriers to participation) was central to the project.

The STATEMENT project was a logical follow-through of an earlier European Union effort, the Horizontal European Activities in Rehabilitation Technology (HEART) report called *Improving Availability of Assistive Technology in Europe*, which recognized that the areas of education, employment, and accessibility are fundamental to the quality of life of people with disabilities and that the availability and provision of ATs have a significant impact on them. The report highlighted the absence of information on the use of ATs in education and in particular at the primary and secondary level, at the same time acknowledging an increased use of ATs, particularly computers, in higher and continuing education. The issues highlighted in the HEART report reflect key questions that need to be addressed in the development of AT services, namely,

- What role can AT play in dismantling barriers faced by students with disabilities in education?

- What factors are important in ensuring the maximum effective use of technology?

- What structures need to be put in place to ensure equality of provision and access to AT?

STATEMENT and the central co-coordinating unit of the project were based in the CTS department of the CRC. The CTS department's primary role was to provide an AT evaluation and advisory service. They utilized an in-depth consultative

Table 7.1. Disability profile of student applicants

Disability	Number	Percent
Hearing impairments	21	25
Learning disabilities	13	15
Mental illness	1	1
Multiple disabilities	6	7
Physical disabilities	39	45
Visual disabilities	6	7
Total	86	100

process, incorporating an experienced evaluation team, the consumer, the consumer's family members, and teachers or other professionals familiar with the consumer's needs. The process is at all stages concerned with empowering the individual in the decision-making process and subsequently empowering him or her to participate more effectively in all aspects of his or her personal life, via the use of AT that may be identified through the evaluation.

Achieving a Student-Centered Evaluation Component

Roulstone (1998) identified ineffective assessment services for AT as being those where

- The primary focus is on the technology provider
- The needs of the provider override those of the person with a disability
- The assessor or provider focuses on disability rather than ability

The STATEMENT project adapted the MPT assessments (Scherer, 1998) as a means of addressing these issues as well as assessing and responding to the individual needs of the students while taking into account the broader factors that lead to a request for assistance and which will likely affect their use or nonuse of technology. The importance of ensuring a person-centered approach and relevant evaluation process is clearly highlighted in the increasing body of research examining AT use by people with disabilities. Specifically, consumers are less likely to use a recommended device when their needs are neither fully addressed nor understood during the technology selection process.

Although the MPT model was developed and evaluated in the United States, the STATEMENT project was the first time in which the model was adapted for use in the Irish context. In particular, the MPT model was adapted to consider the different educational environment and curriculum and different use of language, as well as the different environmental, social, cultural, and personal factors potentially having an impact on the use of technology by students with disabilities. The first months of the project were substantially concerned with researching, developing, and piloting the MPT questionnaires. Figures 7.1, 7.2, and 7.3 are sample

Ireland's Student Matching Person and Technology Form Item 13
View of Disability
How are your current capabilities in the following areas?

Circle the best response for each.

		Poor		Average		Good
A.	Vision	1	2	3	4	5
C.	Speech	1	2	3	4	5
D.	Upper extremity control	1	2	3	4	5
E.	Lower extremity control	1	2	3	4	5
F.	Mobility	1	2	3	4	5
H.	Physical strength/stamina	1	2	3	4	5

Figure 7.1. Sample portion of the Matching Person and Technology form item 13 used in Ireland. In the United States, students are asked to rate each item by placing – beside any items that they believe will weaken over time. They put + next to items they believe will strengthen over time.

portions of the assessment as adapted by the STATEMENT project conducted in the Republic of Ireland (items numbered according to original form).

Through the research, development, and piloting of the MPT model, the STATEMENT project introduced an innovative evaluation tool to support evaluation teams in providing effective evaluation to people with disabilities. The experiences of the STATEMENT project have added significantly to the development of effective assessment tools; to the understanding of the issues that affect the use of technology by students; and to the structures, resource requirements, and challenges inherent in creating person-centered, cost-effective evaluation services,

Ireland's Student Matching Person and Technology Form Item 14
View of Disability/Quality of Life
How are your current capabilities in the following areas?

Directions: Circle the best response for each.

		Not satisfied		Satisfied		Very satisfied
A.	Independent living skills	1	2	3	4	5
C.	Physical comfort and well-being	1	2	3	4	5
F.	Ability to go where desired	1	2	3	4	5
I.	Emotional well-being	1	2	3	4	5

Figure 7.2. Sample portion of the Matching Person and Technology form item 14 used in Ireland. In the United States, students would put a mark next to items they most want to improve over time.

Assessing Individual Needs for Assistive Technology

**Ireland's Student Matching Person and Technology
Form Items Regarding Learning Characteristics**

Circle the number of each statement that describes you.

1. I am curious and excited about new things.
4. I move from task to task easily.
15. I like to try new things.
17. I often want to work slower than others.
24. I am often easily distracted.
26. I am easily bored.
27. I often feel anxious.
33. I sometimes feel intimidated by technology.
34. I prefer to work by myself.

Figure 7.3. Sample portion of the Matching Person and Technology form regarding learning characteristics. This form has the same directions when used in Ireland and the United States.

which ensure the maximum benefit and utilization of technology by people with disabilities. According to the project's final report, "The Matching Person and Technology evaluation piloted as part of the project provided the mechanism for achieving [a client focused evaluation service] and the overwhelming positive reaction from participating students is illustrative of the effectiveness of this approach" (Central Remedial Clinic, 2000, p. iii).

In spite of the positive results, however, the need for further development of the MPT model with advice from people with disabilities and services providers is recognized. Given the delays in students obtaining technology, it has not been possible to comprehensively evaluate the effect of the technology on the educational experience of students. The project has designed a postevaluation questionnaire to assess the effect of technology on the education experience, and the CRC has committed to completing this follow-up.

Key Features for an Effective Assistive Technology Evaluation Service

Overall, the experiences under the STATEMENT project highlight key features required in the development of an effective AT evaluation service. Many of these features, including flexibility, access to training, and ownership, apply in the United States as well as Ireland.

Flexibility

An evaluation service must be flexible enough to respond to the diverse needs of students, diverse environments in which it will operate, and the external factors that may affect it. The MPT preevaluation questionnaire provides an effective mechanism for compiling this information in a systematic and comprehensive way.

Access to Training

An evaluation service must incorporate the following training provisions if a student is to derive maximum benefit from the use of technology:

- Training for the student in use of the AT
- Computer skills training for the student where relevant
- Information and training for the people paying for the AT regarding the technology recommended for the student
- Information and training for educational and training institutions and individual employers regarding the technology recommended for use by the student

Ownership

Despite increased allocation of resources to fund AT, and the substantial role played by AT in supporting access to employment and education by people with disabilities, people with disabilities do not have any recognized entitlement to obtain funding to purchase technology necessary for higher education, training, or employment. Furthermore, no funding or policy is in place to support evaluations of need for technology or training in the use of that technology.[1] All funding agencies should incorporate a clear policy on evaluation of need and training in the use of technology, including a clear strategy for funding and implementation of these services.

Evaluation of Primary and Secondary Students

The STATEMENT project created an awareness of the need for students entering continuing and higher education to be evaluated, but implementing an AT evaluation service for students in primary and secondary schools should be given equal consideration. The consortium of the project are working on a proposal to develop and deliver the service at the secondary school level to ensure that all students who can benefit from the use of AT in education have the opportunity to be evaluated for appropriate technology and to receive ongoing training and support in using that technology.

The experiences of the STATEMENT project have added significantly to the development of effective assessment tools and to the understanding of the issues that impact the use of technology by students. They have also added to the knowledge of the structures, resource requirements, and challenges inherent in creating

---

[1]In the United States, the most common sources for funding include: Medicaid/Medicare, school districts, vocational rehabilitation programs, and Supplemental Security Income/Social Security Disability Insurance.

Table 7.2. Essential steps in the HEART study's evaluation of assistive technology

1. Initiative—the first contact
2. Assessment—evaluation of needs
3. Typology—choosing the appropriate kind of assistive technology
4. Selection—selecting the specific device
5. Authorization—obtaining funding
6. Delivery—getting the device to the user
7. Management—continued help and follow-up for the user

person-centered, cost-effective evaluation services that ensure the maximum benefit and use of technology by people with disabilities. Comparing the "essential steps in evaluation" as recommended by the HEART study (see Table 7.2) with the expanded steps recommended by the STATEMENT project (see Table 7.3) best summarizes this philosophy. The first step in the HEART study assumes that the person with disabilities should take the initiative. The CTS experience is that the service has to be proactive in first giving general information through training, workshops, and so forth on the pros and cons of AT for a given individual. The use of web sites may be one means to accomplish information provision, but it should be supplemented with other means, as it is still the case that many individuals with disabilities do not have access to personal computers.

In keeping with the principles of universal design, more attention should be paid to the usability of devices (Scherer, 2000). People should select technologies based first on how well the technologies satisfy their needs and preferences (Steps 3–5 in Table 7.3), then according to their attractiveness and appeal (Steps 6–10 in

Table 7.3. Essential steps in the STATEMENT project's evaluation of assistive technology

1. Outreach—information workshops/web site information
2. Intake/referral
3. Identification of needs
4. Agreement by all team members on goals
5. Skills evaluation
6. Trial/loan equipment
7. Agree on use/nonuse of assistive technology
8. Fund equipment
9. Train in equipment use
10. Support
11. Follow-up

Table 7.4. Matching Person and Technology components of assistive technology usability

Device evaluation: Assistive technology (AT) meets the individual's functional need
    Milieu: determination of environments in which it will be used
    Person: discussion of preferences and needs
    AT: delineation of desired functions and features

Device selection: AT has appeal and is obtainable
    Milieu: Good device/environment fit exists
    Person: Accepts AT use and is psychologically ready for use
    AT: Product is acceptable in terms of cost, delivery date, aesthetics, and usefulness

Device use: AT performance and achievement of the functional goal
    Milieu: Environmental accommodations in place, AT performs adequately in different environments
    Person: Satisfaction with use
    AT: Has the desired durability and operability

Table 7.3). If it meets the person's performance expectations (Step 11 in Table 7.3) and is easy and comfortable to use, then a good match of person and technology has been achieved. This usability hierarchy can be expressed in terms of the MPT components as shown in Table 7.4.

CONCLUSION

This chapter has described how AT use in school, at home, in the workplace, and in the community has enhanced the available opportunities for people with disabilities in the United States and Ireland to participate in all major life activities. One of the students who participated in STATEMENT and the MPT evaluation process articulated the difference the appropriate technology made in her life:

> Since I received the technology, my life has become unbelievably easier.... Now instead of 3–4 hours it takes me 45 minutes to an hour [to read].... The pressure that I was under is practically gone. For the first time in my life I'm interested and excited about reading and I'm realising how restricted I was... I could never have believed that reading and studying could be this enjoyable. (Central Remedial Clinic, 2000, p. iii–iv)

Although we have described a consumer-centered means for the evaluation and selection of appropriate technologies, much is left undone as far as making technologies available to those who can benefit from their use. Information distribution, adequate training for AT providers and primary and secondary users, and funding need to be given as much priority as the achievement of a good match. The match can be good, but without the means to obtain or best apply the AT, use will be seriously compromised, or worse, won't happen.

REFERENCES

Americans with Disabilities Act (ADA) of 1990, PL 101-336, 42 U.S.C. §§ 12101 *et seq.*
Assistive Technology Act of 1998, PL 105-394, 29 U.S.C. §§ 3001 *et seq.*
Central Remedial Clinic, Republic of Ireland (March 2000). *Evaluation Report, STATEMENT*

Pilot Programme, an EU Horizon Programme project. (Available: http://www.crc.ie/services/technology/projects.htm#statement)

Children's Hospital at Stanford. (1980). *Team effectiveness: A retrospective study.* Palo Alto, CA: Rehabilitation Engineering Center. (NARIC Document No. 03855)

Craddock, G. (2000, March). The mighty Aphrodite. *Proceedings of the 15th Annual International Conference, "Technology and Persons with Disabilities,"* Los Angeles, March 20–25, 2000. [http://www.csun.edu/cod/conf2000/proceedings/0072Craddock.html]

Craddock, G., & Murphy, H.J., (1998). Training under Project Aphrodite. In I. Placencia Porrero & E. Ballabio (Eds.), *Improving the quality of life for the European citizen: Technology for inclusive design & equality.* Amsterdam: 105 Press.

Crewe, N.M., & Dijkers, M. (1995). Functional assessment. In L.C. Cushman & M.J. Scherer (Eds.), *Psychological assessment in medical rehabilitation* (pp. 101–144). Washington, DC: American Psychological Association.

Cushman, L.A., & Scherer, M.J. (1996). Measuring the relationship of assistive technology use, functional status over time, and consumer–therapist perceptions of ATs. *Assistive Technology, 8*(2) 103–109.

European Commission, HEART. (1994). *Improving availability of assistive technology in Europe: Relevance of legal and economic factor.* (Available: http://www.hi.se/english/heart.shtm)

Flemming, J.E., & Flemming, B.P. (1995). *RESNA 1995 Proceedings: Multimedia for Assistive Technology Training and Recruitment: Two CD-ROM Training Programs* (Available http://www.resna.org)

Individuals with Disabilities Education Act (IDEA) of 1990, PL 101-476, 20 U.S.C §§ 1400 *et seq.*

Individuals with Disabilities Education Act (IDEA) Amendments of 1997, PL 105-17, 20 U.S.C. §§ 1400 *et seq.*

Phillips, B., & Zhao, H. (1993). Predictors of assistive technology abandonment. *Assistive Technology, 5,* 36–45.

Rehabilitation Act of 1973, PL 93-112, 29 U.S.C. §§ 701 *et seq.*

Roulstone, A. (1998). *Enabling technology: Disabled people, work, and new technology.* Buckingham, UK: Open University Press.

Scherer, M.J. (1992). *Psychosocial factors associated with the use of technological assistance.* Paper presented at the 100th American Psychological Association Annual Convention, Washington, DC. (ERIC Document Reproduction Service No. ED 350 795)

Scherer, M.J. (1998). *Matching person & technology (MPT) model manual* (3rd ed.). Webster, NY: Institute for Matching Person & Technology.

Scherer, M.J. (2000). *Living in the state of stuck: How technology impacts the lives of people with disabilities* (3rd ed.). Cambridge, MA: Brookline Books.

Scherer, M.J., & Galvin, J.C. (1994). Matching people with technology. *Rehabilitation Management, 9,* 128–130.

Scherer, M.J., & McKee, B. (1990). High-tech communication devices: What separates users from non-users? *Augmentative and Alternative Communication, 6,* 99.

Technology-Related Assistance for Individuals with Disabilities Act of 1988, PL 100-407, 29 U.S.C. §§ 2201 *et seq.*

8

Vocational and Career Assessment

Patricia Rogan, Teresa A. Grossi, and Roberta Gajewski

ELLEN'S CAREER EXPLORATION

Ellen is a 17-year-old high school student who lives with her parents. She wants to go to college, have a job, and live in her own apartment after completing high school. Although Ellen needs assistance in a variety of daily living activities, she has repeatedly proven that her abilities exceed the expectations of the professionals and other adults in her world.

Ellen and her eighth-grade peers began exploring the world of work through career exploration activities in middle school. As a freshman in high school, she began assessing her interests and gathering information about possible jobs she could do. This occurred informally with her parents during family outings, as well as in her career exploration class—a requirement for all freshmen. Also during her freshman year, Ellen received assistance to begin to compile a vocational profile and portfolio.

In the past 3 years, Ellen has continued to learn about her interests and abilities through high school classes, work experiences, and activities with her family and friends outside of school. Her sewing class in school led Ellen to express an interest in working at a fabric store, where later she worked during winter break. With the assistance of her teachers and the transition coordinator, she continues to add information to her profile and portfolio. She currently works part-time as an assistant in the deli at a local supermarket. Ellen would like to graduate next year, move to an apartment, audit classes at the university, and perhaps work part-time in an office environment.

VOCATIONAL ASSESSMENT

Ellen's story represents the evolution of special education, transition services, and school reform efforts in the United States. She has benefited from being included in general education classes, exploring the world of work through a variety of age-appropriate activities with her peers, and developing self-determination skills through active involvement in identifying and recording her interests, goals, and support needs. Details of Ellen's story are provided throughout this chapter.

Work is a central component of a quality adult life. Employment provides a source of income, enhances self-esteem, provides important social connections, and allows people to fulfill their duties as contributing, tax-paying citizens. To be satisfied with their work, it is important that people's jobs match their interests, skills, strengths, and needs. Most people strive to pursue their interests through careers that evolve over time as they build experience, knowledge, and skills. Unfortunately, people with disabilities have been largely left out of the job market. Those who are employed are often in entry-level jobs that may be poorly matched with their interests and skills, with little chance for job expansion and promotion.

Schools play a critical role in preparing youth with disabilities for the world of work. Career exploration and development should begin at an early age and continue through transition to adult life. Students can work to develop positive work attitudes, behaviors, and skills while they take general education classes, participate in integrated extracurricular activities, engage in service learning, work alongside their peers in school jobs, and secure part-time jobs in the community while in high school. All of these activities require a strong assessment process to ensure individualized decisions are made, plans are implemented, and desired outcomes are achieved.

This chapter begins with a brief discussion of current laws that provide guidance to the field in the area of vocational and career assessment. Next, issues with traditional vocational evaluation are highlighted, followed by principles that should underlie vocational assessment. The general process of vocational assessment is delineated next, along with specific types of vocational and career assessment approaches that have proven effective in the transition planning process. The chapter concludes with indicators that might help teams evaluate the success of the process.

Legislation Guiding Vocational Assessment Practices

Based on research outcomes and advice from professionals and consumers, most policy makers recognize that effective assessment is a key component for successful transition, requiring communication, cooperation, and collaboration among stakeholders (Clark, 1998). Quality assessments provide the foundation for all successful special education and transition services (Flexer & Luft, 2001). The Individuals with Disabilities Education Act (IDEA) Amendments of 1997 (PL 105-17) provided a major shift in assessment processes, with a greater emphasis on informal assessments that examine the student's performance within natural environments. The Carl D. Perkins Vocational and Applied Technology Education Act Amendments of 1990 (PL 101-392) mandate that assessments should help facilitate placements in integrated environments and serve as the basis for transition planning and other supports and accommodations for students who receive services under IDEA.

The Rehabilitation Act Amendments of 1992 (PL 102-569) stated that "to the maximum extent appropriate," the use of suitable existing data and information provided by schools, other agencies, and individuals and their families should be used "as a primary source" for making decisions and developing the individualized plan for employment.

The Workforce Investment Act of 1998 (WIA; PL 105-220), of which the Rehabilitation Act of 1998 is a part, provides for One-Stop and Work One Centers designed to provide skill assessment, job training, education, information, and employment services at a single location. All adults age 18 or older, including people with disabilities, have the right to obtain basic or "core" services offered through the Work One Centers. The role of assessment has also been defined in the school-based learning and connecting activities components of the School-to-Work Opportunities Act of 1994 (PL 103-239). All of these pieces of legislation reinforce the importance of assessment and evaluation in the transition process.

Issues with Traditional Vocational Evaluation

Vocational assessment has often been ignored, implemented in a generic fashion, or conducted using inappropriate tools (Parker & Schaller, 1996; Sitlington, Neubert, & Leconte, 1997). Traditional vocational evaluation assumptions and practices have been called into question when applied to people with significant disabilities, including supported employment candidates (Parker & Schaller, 1996; Wehman, 1986). Rogan and Hagner (1990) discussed five of the many problematic features of traditional vocational evaluation procedures.

First, the vocational evaluation process has been used as a screening device to select or reject individuals considered able or unable to benefit from vocational services. The use of vocational evaluation procedures and instruments has resulted in the exclusion of numerous people considered to have significant disabilities from the labor market. A related screening function of traditional vocational evaluation has been to deem some people *job ready* and others not. Those considered *not job ready* have typically been placed in sheltered facilities (Rogan & Hagner, 1990).

Second, traditional vocational evaluations typically occur in artificial, simulated environments such as evaluation centers or sheltered facilities. Individuals may be given a series of psychometric tests, work samples, and in-house situational assessments for the purpose of diagnosis, prediction, and placement (Rudrud, Ziarnik, Bernstein, & Ferrara, 1984). These activities are also largely simulated and artificial, bearing little resemblance to real work in community jobs.

Third, reliability and validity data regarding many traditional assessment tools is absent or lacking (Botterbusch, 1980). Assessment procedures have been used inappropriately with people who have significant disabilities, for whom the instruments were not designed. In addition, unfamiliar tasks, environments, and people contribute to potential problems in reliability and validity (Flexer & Luft, 2001).

Fourth, individuals evaluated within facility-based centers tend to be referred for placement in the very facility in which they were evaluated (Murphy & Hagner, 1988). Economic and organizational forces within the facilities exert a significant influence on evaluation processes and outcomes.

Fifth, vocational evaluations have traditionally occurred as a separate function of the larger job placement and career development efforts. Evaluators are not typically involved with individuals after the assessment has been completed, and little, if any, follow-up information is collected to find out where people were eventually placed or how well they did.

What Guiding Principles Underlie Vocational and Career Assessment?

In response to these problems with traditional vocational evaluations, we offer a set of principles to guide vocational and career assessment. The purpose of vocational assessment is to gather relevant information about each students' strengths, interests, preferences, skills, and needs, with the emphasis on capabilities to assist individuals with disabilities to make informed choices about their future role as a worker and community citizen. The following principles should assist individuals, their families, and school personnel to conduct meaningful vocational assessments:

- Individuals and their family and friends should be involved and empowered to provide information that reflects the individual's history and experiences and to suggest natural, commonsense approaches to employment and career development.

- Varied assessment methods should be selected based on the type of information needed and the experiences and characteristics of each individual, including his or her cultural and linguistic backgrounds.

- Assessments should take place over time. Students should have multiple opportunities to demonstrate their abilities and potential.

- Information should be collected under natural conditions (e.g., in actual environments with actual materials).

- Students should have access to individualized supports, modifications, accommodations, and/or assistive technology to enhance their performance and to fully demonstrate his or her true abilities and potential.

- The focus should be on successful functioning in integrated environments with the necessary services and supports brought in, rather than the person having to fit the environment. Assessment activities are *not* used to deem a person unemployable, to exclude students from integrated opportunities, or to engage students in meaningless readiness activities that bear no resemblance to real work.

What Is the Process of Vocational Assessment?

As Callahan and Garner (1997) stated, the starting point of vocational services is discovery of who the people really are behind the veil of disability, what they want, and what they might be able to contribute to employers. Individuals, parents, and professionals should begin the vocational assessment process with a presumption of employability. Vocational assessment follows the same process of person-centered planning described in other chapters. Although there are variations in approaches, general components include the following:

- Invite people who work most closely with the individual and who know the individual best to participate as members of the team.
- Start with the end in mind by assisting the individual to describe personal goals and desired outcomes and by seeking input from people who know the student best.
- Describe the student's current situation and what is already known about him or her.
- Identify necessary information that is important for planning next steps, and decide how best to gather such information.
- Gather and document needed information.
- Develop short-term and long-term action steps that will lead to desired outcomes. Include timelines and people responsible.
- Translate this information into the student's individualized transition plan (ITP).
- Evaluate progress and intermediate outcomes on an ongoing basis.
- Revise and update the action plan as needed.
- Develop a longitudinal record (e.g., portfolio) to document vocational/career development activities, accomplishments, outcomes, and other artifacts that will assist adult service providers.

WHAT VOCATIONAL AND CAREER ASSESSMENT APPROACHES MIGHT BE USED?

There are many informal (functional) and formal (standardized) assessment approaches that have been developed and used for vocational and career assessment. Table 8.1 provides a listing of various assessment approaches.

Functional, or informal, assessments typically focus on practical skills in current or future environments. Functional assessments share some of the following characteristics. They 1) focus on practical, independent living and work skills that enable the person to survive and succeed in the real world; 2) have an ecological emphasis on the person's performance or behavior in specific environments; 3) examine the process of learning and performance; 4) suggest intervention techniques that may be successful; and 5) specify procedures for monitoring and evaluating student progress (Gaylord-Ross & Browder, 1991, p. 45). Some examples of functional assessment approaches include vocational profiles, observations, interviews and questionnaires, ecological interventions and workplace analyses, situational assessments, curriculum-based assessments, and portfolio assessments. Each of these is discussed next.

Standardized, or formal, assessments are designed to determine an individual's relative standing for a particular trait or characteristic in relation to a norm

Table 8.1. Approaches for gathering assessment information

Method	Description
Interviews and questionnaires	Interviews with students, family members, former teachers, friends, counselors, other support staff, and former employers
Observations	Observations of the student within typical daily environments and activities
Ecological and environmental inventories	Inventories involve gathering information about specific geographic areas (e.g., neighborhoods) or environments (e.g., workplaces)
Situational assessment	Observing and assessing the student's behaviors in environments that will closely resemble his or her future working, living, or educational environments
Curriculum-based vocational assessment	An approach conducted 1) during program placement to determine the appropriateness of the placement and the type of support services needed, 2) during participation in the vocational program to assess the progress, and 3) during program exiting to determine support services needed to transition into employment and/or post-secondary education
Interest inventories	Interest inventories are typically paper-and-pencil instruments that solicit information about personal and occupational preferences
Vocational profile	A compilation of relevant work-related information gathered through interactions with the individual and others who know the person, inventories of the person's neighborhood, and observations of the individual in a variety of settings
Portfolio assessment	Includes samples of the student's behavior over time, collected using multiple procedures (e.g., written products, videotape). The sample tasks are regularly performed in the natural environment in which the student participates to the degree possible in selecting materials to be included.

group. Examples often used for special education and transition programs include vocational and career aptitude, interest, and occupational skills tests. Standardized tests have been criticized for focusing on deficits, providing a narrow and limited view of the individual, and having problems with reliability and validity, especially for individuals with disabilities (Flexer & Luft, 2001).

The type of vocational assessment approach to use depends on the type of information being sought. For example, vocational assessment activities for middle school–age students may focus on the students' knowledge of various career clusters and their understanding of their interests and support needs. Assessments for high school–age students may seek information about student interests, strengths, likes and dislikes, and support needs or about specific classes or experiences the student had (or would like to have). For students in transition, assessments may focus on specific job skills and behaviors, actual jobs that the student will continue postschool, or postsecondary education and training options.

VOCATIONAL PROFILES

The individualized nature of person-centered assessment and planning mandates that employment and other career development activities be structured around individuals rather than individuals being "placed" into existing programs or slots. This people-first rather than program-first or job-first orientation requires that team members responsible for assisting the individual get to know him or her. Although this premise appears obvious, it has often been overlooked (Rogan & Hagner, 1990).

A vocational profile is like "a picture of the individual painted in words" (Callahan & Garner, 1997, p. 99). It is a compilation of information gathered through interactions with the individual and others who know the person, inventories of the person's neighborhood, and observations of the individual in a variety of environments. Each of these methods will be described in this section. Vocational profiles generally address the following information:

- Identification information (e.g., name, address, telephone number, date of birth, marital status)

- Residential/domestic information (e.g., current living situation, including people with whom the individual lives, residential history, family support available, typical routines, friends and social groups, description and location of neighborhood, transportation available, services near home, specific employers near home)

- Educational information (e.g., general history and performance, vocational classes and experiences, community-based instruction and performance)

- Work experience information (e.g., volunteer and informal work performed at home, school, and/or in the community; paid work experiences)

- Current skills across life domains (e.g., performance in home living, community, leisure, social, academic, motor/mobility, communication, other areas of daily living)

- Learning and performance characteristics (e.g., successful teaching and learning approaches, nature of support typically needed, methods that should be avoided, environmental conditions that work best)

- Interests and preferences (e.g., activities that the individual most enjoys and is good at, types of jobs the individual would prefer)

- Connections (e.g., personal contacts of the individual, family, friends, school staff, potential employment leads)

- Accommodations that may be needed in the workplace (e.g., possible adaptations, accessibility issues, accommodations, and personal supports that may be needed at work)

Vocational profile information should be compiled in a clear, concise format using positive language that portrays the person with dignity and respect. Jargon and labels should be avoided. With this information, the team has a strong base for supporting the individual to make choices and decisions about next steps. If employment is desired, specific types of employment and actual employers in the area can be targeted, and plans for contacts should be made.

Observations Across Environments, Activities, and People

The obvious place to start in any assessment activity is with the focal individual and those who know the person best. One way to get to know someone is simply to spend time with him or her in a variety of daily activities and environments. For example, a transition coordinator might meet a student in the student's home, accompany the student to lunch at a restaurant, and/or spend leisure time together. Through these observations and interactions, information about the student's likes and dislikes, behaviors in various settings, social/communication, motor/mobility, transportation, functional academic skills, and support needs can be gathered.

The transition coordinator spent most of her time observing Ellen in her classroom and at her community-based instruction (e.g., grocery shopping, using the local library and bank). The coordinator was able to observe that Ellen had a warm, outgoing personality. With this type of information, work experience opportunities where Ellen could interact with people were pursued.

Interviews and Questionnaires with Students and Family Members

There are a variety of formats for gathering and recording information from students and family members. Student and parent or guardian questionnaires or surveys are often used. Sample student and parent or guardian questions are listed in Table 8.2 and 8.3.

If students and their parents or guardians can read and write, they can complete the questionnaires at their leisure at home; however, it is helpful to use these questionnaires as an interview guide for the teacher or transition coordinator. In this way, follow-up questions can be asked to clarify or expand on given information.

Interviews and questionnaires can also be developed for other team members and people who know the student (e.g., peers, neighbors, counselors, teachers).

Table 8.2. Sample student survey questions

What kind of work or education do you see yourself doing after high school?
What type of work experiences have you had?
What part of the work experiences did you enjoy? Not enjoy?
What do you do for fun?
Who do you hang out with?
Where do you see yourself living after high school or a few years later?
What kind of activities do you participate in now (e.g., church, sports)?
Are there things you hope to start doing in the future (e.g., join a club, get active in political groups, vote)?
How do you get around (transportation)?

Table 8.3. Sample parent or guardian survey questions

What kind of work or education do you see your child doing after high school?
What type of work experiences has your child had over the last few years?
What part of the work experiences do you think he or she enjoyed? Did not enjoy?
What does your child do for fun?
Who does your child spend time with?
Where do you see your child living after high school or a few years later?
What kinds of activities does your child participate in now (e.g., church, sports)?
Are there things you hope your child will start doing in the future (e.g., join a club, get active in a political group, vote)?
How does your child get around (transportation)?

Open-ended questions often elicit rich, in-depth information, as opposed to yes-or-no or forced-choice questions.

Verbal interview formats require sophisticated communication and introspection skills that not all students possess. In such cases, alternative communication formats must be used and/or other methods of information gathering should be pursued.

Although interviews and questionnaires can reap important information, it is important for school personnel to avoid overburdening students and families each year with the same forms and questions. In addition, family members should be asked how they would like to give and receive information.

Ellen's first transition planning meeting at age 14 was held informally at her house with her parents and her teacher. They all talked in general about what Ellen might want to do when she graduated. They also talked about what might be some vocational activities Ellen could participate in at the high school to help her acquire some job skills. While Ellen and her parents knew that Ellen wanted a job after high school, they were not sure at the time which type of job. As Ellen progressed in school, her parents were asked to complete a survey each year indicating not only domains but also suggesting possible courses. With the information from the survey and Ellen's selection of course electives, the IEP team was better able to find some suitable work experience.

Neighborhood Inventory

Decisions about postschool employment must make sense in relation to where an individual lives. Proximity to home and access to viable transportation options are typically high priorities for people with disabilities. Thus, the individual's home should be viewed as the center for job development and other community-based vocational and career development activities.

A neighborhood inventory involves assessing the array of businesses and other community activities and resources within a reasonable distance of an individual's home. Information about aspects such as accessibility, hours of operation, costs, services being offered, and clientele will assist with decisions about jobs, recreation and social activities, adult education options, and personal services. This information can be easily gathered by walking or driving around the student's neighborhood. If an alternate living situation is being sought for the student prior to or soon after the student exits school, it is important to focus on this neighborhood.

A close friend of Ellen's helped her to drive around the community to see if there were any places she might like to work. They also considered the issue of Ellen getting to and from work. Since there was no public transportation available in the community, emphasis was given to finding a job that Ellen could reach by walking or taking a taxi from the apartment she had planned to move to.

Ecological Inventories and Workplace Analysis

In addition to gathering information about students and their neighborhoods, it is important to learn about the environments in which the student will learn (e.g., vocational education classes, postsecondary education) or work (e.g., jobsites). This type of information is needed to assess the person–environment–activity match that is so crucial to success. Too often, individuals with disabilities were placed in training situations or jobs that did not match their interests, skills, and support needs. When the situation falls apart, the individual is often deemed a failure. In reality, the success of an individual with a disability rests largely on the ability of the environment to build on the person's unique gifts and accommodate the person's support needs. For these reasons, environmental assessments are critical in the assessment process.

One method for gathering relevant information about an environment is to conduct an ecological inventory or workplace analysis. Ecological assessments have been commonly used with students who have significant disabilities, but can be useful with all students with disabilities. Information about the physical environment (accessibility, layout), typical activities or work tasks (including rate, sequence, quality, frequency, duration), people therein (age, gender, characteristics of supervisors and co-workers, nature of interactions), and climate or culture (customs, traditions, rituals, routines, rules, expectations) can be gathered through observations and interactions with people who work there. Table 8.4 provides a framework for an ecological inventory.

Table 8.4. Framework for an ecological assessment

Identify the targeted environment (e.g., insurance company, hospital, retail store). Describe environmental conditions (e.g., lighting, layout, accessibility, number of co-workers and proximity, dress code, chain of command)

Determine the sub-environments where the student will be required to perform the skills (e.g., admissions department).

Identify the activities the student will be required to perform (e.g., answering the phone, taking the intake information).

List the skills for each of the activities the student will be required to perform (e.g., interacting with customers, filing forms).

Record student performance in work routines and social interactions.

Analyze discrepancies between student performance and expectations.

Determine interventions and strategies to improve student performance.

Although Ellen indicated a strong desire to secure a job in a bank, the local branches did not have positions open that matched Ellen's skills. Seeking to find a job that Ellen might like, the transition coordinator took note of Ellen's familiarity with the local supermarket (she knew the layout of the store by memory); her friendly smile, which matched the store's current ad slogan; the store's commitment to hiring and supporting individuals with disabilities; the availability of transportation via a taxi; and the many opportunities for job expansion. With that in mind, Ellen's bagging pace picked up, and with her winning smile and personality, Ellen succeeded in receiving a number of letters of recognition of good service from customers. She has since gone on to work in the cheese department, where she continues to enjoy her environment and her job.

Situational Assessments

Another method of gathering relevant information about a student in the context of specific work environments is through the use of situational assessments. Situational assessments entail systematic observation of an individual in a real environment such as a community workplace. Situational assessments have been used for years to introduce students to various work environments and tasks, to gather relevant information about a student's general work skills, and to invite community employers to open their doors to employment opportunities for youth with disabilities.

There are pros and cons to using situational assessments. For many students, actually trying out a job in a real business environment provides tangible information for decision making. The student gains valuable insights about whether he or she likes that particular type of work; however, because each business is unique, performing work in one environment may not provide a complete picture of that career area. Also, because situational assessments provide only a "snapshot" of the student, decisions about the student's skills and potential must be made cautiously.

In practice, situational assessments may last from several hours to several days. Individuals are introduced to a specific work area, work tasks, and co-workers and perform the designated work for the negotiated period of time. The work may be paid or volunteer, depending on the purpose, duration, and skills of the individual.

In high school, Ellen was given the opportunity to select general education courses of interest and to gain work experience in job settings that matched her interest and needs. Ellen had an interest in clothes, so the vocational coordinator set up a situational assessment at a local department store. Ellen worked in the dressing rooms organizing clothes, returning clothes to their proper racks, and keeping the rooms orderly. Albeit brief, this situational assessment enabled the job coach to observe her positive interactions with employees and customers, her work skills, and her good work ethic. This experience led Ellen to take a sewing class in school and secure a job at a fabric store.

Curriculum-Based Assessment

Curriculum-based assessment provides information about a student's progress on specific activities and objectives within an academic or vocational curriculum.

This approach also allows an analysis of the curriculum itself in order to break it down into smaller objectives or tasks. Curriculum-based assessments can also use criterion-referenced measures reflecting specific real-world expectations or standards. For example, a cosmetology curriculum expects the same performance standards as state examiners.

Portfolio Assessment

Portfolios are comprised of evidence of student activities and accomplishments. Portfolios can be very helpful in the transition process and can include documentation of student work experiences, job-related skills, employer evaluations and recommendations, work samples, academic performance, and social skills. Students can be directly involved in developing their portfolios and assessing their growth and development (Carey, 1994; Sarkees-Wircenski & Wircenski, 1994). Videotapes of students with disabilities working in community jobs can provide convincing evidence to prospective employers.

Interest Inventories

Interest inventories are paper-and-pencil instruments that solicit information about personal and occupational preferences. A variety of commercially developed interest inventories exist, such as the Strong Interest Inventory (Hanson, 1985) and the Kuder DD Occupational Interest Survey (Zytowski, 1985). Because some of these measures have not been developed or standardized on populations of students with disabilities, the use of career interest inventories has been discouraged (Clark, Unger, & Stewart, 1993). What's more, many youth have not had enough experience to make valid responses regarding their career goals and aspirations.

In summary, there are a wide array of assessment approaches for transition planning and evaluation. Some of the more commonly used methods are described here. The more time and effort put into vocational assessment activities, the better the quality of information; however, because students are often over-assessed in school, it is important to be selective and focused when choosing and conducting assessment activities.

How Might Teams Evaluate the Success of the Process?

Assessment and evaluation processes must be ongoing in order to determine the success of particular actions and outcomes. It is imperative that both the individual vocational outcomes and the overall program effectiveness are evaluated. This information can provide areas of need for the student as well as areas for program improvement. The ultimate goal of services must result in meaningful outcomes for the student. There are a number of areas of information that should be gathered to address the success of the process.

Vocational and Career Assessment

Student Satisfaction

The performance, satisfaction, and social acceptance of the student should be monitored periodically over time to determine if the activities, settings, and supports continue to be a good match for the person. Job satisfaction is an important component of career development. It is no surprise that job dissatisfaction correlates with job loss, absenteeism, and interpersonal problems (Dawis, 1984). There are a number of questions that can be asked to determine if the student was satisfied with the services. These and other similar questions could be asked as open-ended questions or using a Likert scale (e.g., 1=never, 5=always). For example,

- Did the staff get to know you before and during the process, including your strengths, likes, dislikes, and needs?
- Were you involved in the decision making of the activities?
- Were you involved in determining how you learn best and what teaching methods work better for you?
- Were choices given to you throughout the process?
- When on the job sites, did the staff represent your interests as best as possible?
- Did the staff help you to get to know your co-workers?
- Were services provided in a timely manner?
- Do you enjoy the type of work you are doing?
- Do you understand what is expected of you at your job?
- Are you happy with the number of hours you are working?
- Are you happy with the pay you are receiving from your work?

Additional information should be gathered from family members, businesses, and agencies regarding their satisfaction with the program or services.

Ellen's first work experience was in a cafeteria at a nursing home. Since the school had cafeteria jobs as their initial placements and since Ellen liked people, the job developer decided that the nursing home might be a good placement. After a few weeks of successful employment, Ellen began to lose interest. Believing that the cafeteria job was a good match and uncertain about the nursing home environment, the job developer switched Ellen to an elementary school cafeteria. Once again, Ellen's initial performance was satisfactory, and her enthusiasm indicated that this might be a successful placement; however, after a few weeks, she began to lose interest. Through careful observation at the job site and discussion with her family, it was noted that Ellen did not like washing dishes, nor did she like cleaning tables. It became obvious that her dislikes for those particular chores outweighed her desire to work with people.

With the desire to build Ellen's self-confidence, efforts were made to find a summer job for her that would capitalize on some of her other interests. Knowing that Ellen wanted to work in an office and have her own "name plate," her transition team was able to secure a job at a large, local realty company. With the help of the job developer, they were able to carve a position where she could prepare mailings for the various realtors. The job enabled Ellen to hone her job skills, practice social skills, and learn travel transportation skills (because she had to take a taxicab home). This placement was successful and set a precedent for Ellen.

Student Outcomes

There are a number of factors that should be assessed to determine the student outcomes. How well special education and transition programs prepare students for adult life is often determined by what they are doing beyond high school. Recent federal and state legislation and policies have reinforced the need to obtain information on former students who received special education services. This information will inform legislators, policy makers, administrators, school personnel, and family members about the effectiveness of the programs and services. Graduate follow-up information should reflect one's life space as well as the services and supports in place. Information to be gathered may include employment (e.g., wages, hours worked per week, benefits, type of work, integration level, transportation), community living (e.g., type of living situation, number of roommates, level of support needed, degree of choice and control), social/leisure (e.g., nature of social networks, type of recreation/leisure activities, frequency of using community services, degree of support needed, degree of freedom), and postsecondary education (e.g., type of postsecondary program or school, area of study, projected date of completion).

Program Outcomes

To support successful student outcomes, a number of program elements should be in place. Some of these elements include sufficient numbers of well-trained staff, access to inclusive programs and services, the provision of individualized adaptations and accommodations, access to typical transportation options, and sufficient funding and administrative support. Without these in place, student services and outcomes are likely to suffer.

CONCLUSION

The process of transition planning, service delivery, and evaluation begins with and builds on ongoing assessment information. The ultimate goal of transition assessment activities is to gather relevant information about each student and his or her aspirations, strengths, interests, preferences, and needs in order to plan and provide appropriate activities, services, and supports. By using a variety of assessment approaches, a comprehensive profile can be developed and team members can feel confident that desired outcomes will be achieved.

REFERENCES

Botterbusch, K. (1980). *A comparison of vocational evaluation systems*. Menomonie: University of Wisconsin–Stout, Materials Development Center.
Callahan, M.J., & Garner, J.B. (1997). *Keys to the workplace: Skills and supports for people with disabilities*. Baltimore: Paul H. Brookes Publishing Co.
Carey, L. (1994). *Measuring and evaluating school learning*. Boston: Allyn & Bacon.
Carl D. Perkins Vocational and Applied Technology Education Act Amendments of 1990, PL 101-392, 104 Statutes at Large 753–804, 806–834.
Clark, G.M. (1998). *Assessment for transition planning*. Austin, TX: PRO-ED.
Clark, H., Unger, K., & Stewart, E. (1993). Transition of youth and young adults with emotional/behavioral disorders into employment, education, and independent living. *Community Alternatives: International Journal of Family Care, 5*(2), 19–46.
Dawis, R. (1984). Job satisfaction: Worker aspirations, attitudes, and behavior. In N. Gysbers & Associates (Eds.), *Designing careers* (pp. 275–302). San Francisco, CA: Jossey-Bass.
Flexer, R., & Luft, P. (2001). Transition assessment and post school outcomes. In R. Flexer, T. Simmons, P. Luft, & R. Baer (Eds.), *Transition planning for secondary students with disabilities* (pp. 197–226). Upper Saddle River, NJ: Prentice Hall.
Gaylord-Ross, R., & Browder, D. (1991). Functional assessment: Dynamic and domain properties. In L.H. Meyer, C.A. Peck, & L. Brown (Eds.), *Critical issues in the lives of people with severe disabilities*. Baltimore: Paul H. Brookes Publishing Co.
Hanson, J. (1985). *User's guide for the Strong Interest Inventory* (Rev. ed.). Stanford, CA: Stanford University Press.
Individuals with Disabilities Education Act (IDEA) Amendments of 1997, PL 105-17, 20 U.S.C. §§ 1400 *et seq.*
Individuals with Disabilities Education Act (IDEA) of 1990, PL 101-476, 20 U.S.C. §§ 1400 *et seq.*
Murphy, S., & Hagner, D. (1988). Evaluation assessment settings: Ecological influences on vocational evaluation. *Journal of Rehabilitation, 53,* 53–59.
Parker, R., & Schaller, J. (1996). Issues in vocational assessment and disability. In E. Szymanski & R. Parker (Eds.), *Work and disability: Issues and strategies in career development and job placement* (pp. 127–164). Austin, TX: PRO-ED.
Rehabilitation Act Amendments of 1992, PL 102-569, 29 U.S.C. §§ 701 *et seq.*
Rogan, P., & Hagner, D. (1990). Vocational evaluation in supported employment. *Journal of Rehabilitation, 56*(1), 45–57.
Rudrud, E.H., Ziarnik, J.P., Bernstein, G.S., & Ferrara, J.M. (1984). *Proactive vocational habilitation*. Baltimore: Paul H. Brookes Publishing Co.
Sarkees-Wircenski, M., & Wircenski, J. (1994). Transition planning: Developing a career portfolio for students with disabilities. *Career Development for Exceptional Individuals, 17,* 203–214.
School-to-Work Opportunities Act of 1994, PL 103-239, 20 U.S.C. §§ 6101 *et seq.*
Sitlington, P., Neubert, D., & LeConte, P. (1997). Transition assessment: The position of the Division of Career Development and Transition. *Career Development for Exceptional Individuals, 20*(1), 69–79.
Wehman, P. (1986). Supported competitive employment for persons with severe disabilities. *Journal of Applied Rehabilitation Counseling, 17,* 24–29.
Workforce Investment Act (WIA) of 1998, PL 105-220, 29 U.S.C. §§ 794d.
Zytowski, D. (1985). *Kuder DD Occupational Interest Survey [manual supplement]*. Chicago: Science Research Associates.

9

Transition Service Integration Model

Ensuring that the Last Day of School Is No Different from the Day After

Nicholas J. Certo, Caren L. Sax, Ian Pumpian,
Denise Mautz, Kimberly A. Smalley, Holly A. Wade, and David A. Noyes

TRANSITION TO WHAT?

Jaime began working at the grocery store near his high school when he turned 19. The grocery store served as an unpaid vocational training site for many students as part of their career path exploration. Students expanded their work experience by trying a variety of jobs including bagging groceries, stocking shelves, working in the produce department, returning "go-backs" (items that customers decide not to purchase), and working as a cashier. Jaime, who used a manual wheelchair and was labeled with a cognitive disability, liked the grocery business. His family shopped at this store regularly, so he knew many of the employees. Jaime enjoyed the bustling activity that typically occurred in the store, and he quickly learned that there were always things that needed to be done. His teacher designed a picture chart showing the layout of the store, making it easier to learn where everything belonged. Jaime often referred to his picture-coded list of things to do that remained attached to his wheelchair with a clip and a handy carrying case. Jaime started out in a training position, working fewer than 5 hours a week. As he became more familiar with the store routine, his co-workers and bosses, and the variety of responsibilities, he wanted to work more hours; however, it was time for Jaime to move to the next

---

Preparation of this manuscript was supported in part by grants from the U.S. Department of Education, Office of Special Education Programs (Grant # H078C60008; Grant # H158Q70009), and Rehabilitative Services Administration (Grant # H235W70045). No official endorsement should be inferred.

By *significant disabilities,* we are referring to individuals with moderate to profound intellectual disabilities, some of whom also have secondary sensory or physical disabilities.

work experience site, leaving the grocery world behind. The series of jobs available to the students were designated as training sites; therefore, they were not often available to the students beyond the work experience period. Even if the employer wanted to hire Jaime directly, there was no guarantee that the support Jaime required would continue.

By the time Jaime was ready to exit school at age 22, he had experienced high points and low points at a number of jobsites. His transition teacher arranged for a planning meeting in April (he was scheduled to graduate in June) and invited Jaime's family, the case service coordinator from the department of developmental disabilities, and a representative from the department of rehabilitation. All of the parties involved agreed that supported employment was an appropriate goal for Jaime, so an application was made for vocational rehabilitation services. Because the application process and eligibility determination for rehabilitation services can take up to 60 days, Jaime and his family were encouraged to visit adult agencies to discuss supported employment options and to decide who would provide the best services for Jaime to find and maintain employment.

By June, rehabilitation services were authorized for Jaime, and an adult agency began to provide job development and identify an appropriate employment match. Jaime exited school and stayed at home until a job was identified. After 2 months of waiting, Jaime was offered a job at a sheltered workshop until a community placement could be found. Jaime and his family refused this option, feeling that this was a step backward, as he was working successfully in the community while he was in school. Two more months passed, leaving Jaime bored and his family frustrated. Momentum and motivation were lost.

WHAT ARE THE OUTCOMES?

Jaime's story helps to illustrate a critical issue in transition planning. Due to delayed interagency collaboration and planning, too many students experience this "black hole" at the end of their school career. Much of the progress many students make during their school-based work experiences in the community is interrupted at the time of transition. Traditionally, students exit school transition programs at age 22 and are referred to an appropriate adult agency (i.e., a nonprofit program providing services for people with disabilities in the community). In general, students like Jaime must leave current employment because it is part of the school training program used by all classmates. The exiting student typically has to start over with unfamiliar program staff, begin a new job with a job coach, and try to establish relationships with new co-workers. Any natural supports that had been developed at the jobsite are forfeited. Is this unusual? Why does this happen? Is there a better way?

Ask any teacher who's been involved in the process of supporting students exiting from the somewhat protective cocoon of special education services in high school into the unknown world of adult life, and they are likely to share a story or two similar to Jaime's. The statistics demonstrating student outcomes have not been encouraging. The National Council on Disability (NCD) and Social Security Administration (SSA) published a report in November 2000 on the transition and postschool outcomes for youth with disabilities regarding employment and education (NCD/SSA, 2000). Of the 6 million students who receive services under the Individuals with Disabilities Education Act (IDEA) of 1990 (PL 101-476) and its subsequent amendments, almost 45% are in secondary school programs. The total number of U.S. students from 18 to 24 years old is increasing and expected to rise at least through 2010; however, appropriate services do not appear to be keeping step with the needs.

Only 25% of students with mental retardation and 15% of those with multiple disabilities are employed 2 years after school exit (Blackorby & Wagner, 1996). This number rises slightly to 37% and 17% respectively 3–5 years after exit (Wagner & Blackorby, 1996). In addition, these same individuals are at greater risk for poverty (Butterworth & Gilmore, 2000; La Plante, Kennedy, Kaye, & Wenger, 1996) because many rely solely on cash benefits from federal income support programs, which are substantially below the poverty level (NCD/SSA, 2000). For example, Affleck, Edgar, Levine, and Kortering (1990) reported that more than 90% of special education graduates are living below the poverty level 3 years after graduation. When this finding is compared with the 2001 unemployment figures of 70% (Bush, 2001), it is clear that the high unemployment and subsequent poverty rates of graduates of special education systems have remained unchanged for decades.

The incidence of students with disabilities attending postsecondary institutions does not fare much better. A survey of about 155,000 freshman college students (NCD/SSA, 2000) indicated that 1 in 11 first-time full-time students self-reported a disability. Disabilities were described related to hearing, speech, orthopedic, learning, health-related, partially sighted or blind, or other conditions. Families of students with significant disabilities have been examining postsecondary options for their sons and daughters who have not traditionally attended college. An electronic listserv was created in response to this need, hosted by the Institute on Disability in New Hampshire. Judging from the inquiries and stories from families nationwide regarding access to postsecondary education, the number of students attending colleges and universities is extremely low, and the strategies for gaining access point to individual advocacy versus any systematic approach. Attitudinal barriers and other disincentives exist, keeping this number low. Problems include confusion about how to obtain resources for reasonable accommodations and whose responsibility it is to cover these costs.

Sadly, this situation has occurred despite attempts via legislation to address the needs of students exiting the public school system. Transition planning is explicitly mandated in the IDEA Amendments of 1997 (PL 105-17), the Rehabilitation Act Amendments of 1992 (PL 102-569), School-to-Work Opportunities Act of 1994 (PL 103-239), and state developmental disabilities legislation (e.g., Lanterman Developmental Disabilities Services Act of 1976, as amended in California) in which integrated employment, postsecondary education, and independent living are expected outcomes. Furthermore, public schools spend close to a quarter of a million dollars on each graduate with significant disabilities during the 19 or more years they are enrolled; however, the rehabilitation or developmental disabilities systems often start over to design services for these graduates (Certo, Pumpian, Fisher, Storey, & Smalley, 1997). This is a significant expenditure with questionable personal and societal benefits. Lastly, despite the rise in normalized educational experiences through inclusive school-based programs (e.g., Fisher, Sax, & Pumpian, 1999), most graduates with significant disabilities still are served primarily in sheltered, segregated environments with limited access to normalized community environments (Mank, 1994; McGaughey, Kiernan, McNally, & Gilmore, 1995; Wehman & West, 1996). It is difficult to imagine that individuals who have experienced inclusion in school will continue to accept less than full inclusion into society at large after exiting school.

WHY HAS THE LEGISLATION BEEN INEFFECTIVE?

Based on federal and state law, three publicly funded service systems—special education, rehabilitation, and developmental disabilities—have separate, but essentially equal, responsibility for the same outcome for transition of youth with significant disabilities. The responsibilities include transition into integrated paid employment, as well as supporting transition into inclusive nonwork community activities (e.g., recreation, community living, postsecondary education). In spite of the investment of time, effort, and public money since the early 1990s, unemployment, congregate living, and lack of access to postsecondary education have remained widespread national problems for individuals with significant disabilities (Mank, 1994; McGaughey et al., 1995; U.S. Bureau of the Census, 1992; Wehman, Revell, & Kregel, 1997).

A major contributing factor to these dismal outcomes is likely the artificial separation maintained by the special education, rehabilitation, and developmental disabilities systems. This separation creates two basic service delivery dilemmas. The first dilemma is limited funding within each system and the chronic understaffing that results.

A LOOK AT THE THREE SYSTEMS

Let's look at each of the three systems. The *special education system* in public schools has not demonstrated its ability to meet its responsibilities in this separated tri-agency delivery system. Acquiring general and specific job skills, securing employment, maintaining employment, and establishing a career for an individual with significant disabilities is a long-term, labor-intensive activity (Pumpian, Fisher, Certo, & Smalley, 1997). Given all of the financial demands on public schools, it is difficult to adequately staff career placement services. These services are additional to a student's basic educational program, including a range of career exploration and development services delivered prior to the student's final year.

The *rehabilitation system* has not demonstrated its ability to meet its responsibilities in this separated tri-agency delivery system. Rehabilitation has had a tendency to serve less challenging, easier-to-place individuals and views job placement as a terminal step rather than the beginning step in the development of a career. This is largely a result of scarce funds, traditional training and practice, and an implicit policy incorporated into the Rehabilitation Act Amendments that employment support is a temporary need. This implicit policy, along with limited funding has resulted in limiting the duration of services (Pumpian et al., 1997; Szymanski, Hanley-Maxwell, & Asselin, 1992). Individuals with significant disabilities often are employed in businesses that are most affected by market forces, which lead to layoffs and the need for retraining (Wehman, 2001).

Furthermore, the fact that the support needs of this population fluctuate unpredictably over time is at variance with the rehabilitation practice of decreasing supported employment services. Individuals with significant disabilities are less likely to be successful or advance in their careers in a system where job placement is a terminal step. As a result, rehabilitation-funded vendors find it difficult to provide integrated employment services to more individuals with significant disabilities even though services to these individuals have been a priority in the rehabilitation system since 1986.

The *developmental disabilities service system (DDS)* has not demonstrated its ability to meet its responsibilities in this separated tri-agency delivery system. This system does have the flexibility to provide long-term support, making successful employment a realistic possibility. Unfortunately, this system still is dominated by programs that adhere to a readiness model that sustains segregated facilities. For example, McGaughey and colleagues (1995) found a 28% increase in segregated programs for individuals with significant disabilities from 1986 to 1991. Furthermore, existing providers have little incentive and support for converting their services to provide integrated employment and community outcomes. There are limited funds available for new services and new provider start-ups to meet this service demand. In other words, the DDS has not been able, under our current separated delivery system, to create a market incentive to "convert" the segregated facility-based programs that dominate the system to meet the integrated outcomes implicit in the agencies legislated authority (McGaughey et al., 1995; Wehman, Revell, & Kregel, 1997).

The second dilemma is the logistical and continuity difficulties created when one system (e.g., the public school) provides instructional experiences and develops job placements and related support skills and another system (e.g., a rehabilitation or developmental disabilities vendor) is required to maintain the placement. Physically helping an individual make the transition across systems and agencies presents such issues as 1) finding a receiving agency with openings in June or July when the school year ends, 2) securing a job placement that meets the individual's interests and needs and can be effectively supported first by school and then by receiving agency staff, and 3) making adequate meeting time available for all staff involved.

When one looks at the collective participation of all three systems, it seems that more than enough funds, staff, and technical expertise are already available to significantly affect the postschool problems frequently lamented in the literature (e.g., Mank 1994; Wehman, West, Kregel, & Kane-Johnson, 1997). Clearly, what is needed is a unified effort by all three service systems that are equally, but independently, responsible for transition. Services must be restructured by sharing responsibility and redirecting joint resources into an integrated short-term, one-stop system at the point of transition, that is, the final year a youth with significant disabilities is in public school.

A NEW WAY OF DOING BUSINESS

Many states have implemented a variety of approaches to address these issues (Kohler & Hood, 2000). One approach that focuses on increasing communication and collaboration across the three systems (e.g., schools, developmental disabilities, rehabilitation) is the Transition Service Integration Model (TSIM; Pumpian & Certo, 1996–1999), implemented in California since 1997. Joint investment clears the path for a seamless transition from school to competitive employment and an integrated adult life. Employment services and job accommodations in inclusive job environments can be established prior to graduation and continued and enhanced without interruption in order to maintain and expand these employment and community access outcomes throughout adulthood (Certo et al., 1997). The remainder of this chapter explains how the model operates, presents a summary of accomplishments, and offers implications for others wishing to implement this approach.

We, along with many participants, have developed and implemented TSIM in approximately a dozen communities in California. Application of the model has resulted in a seamless transition from school to adult life including the following outcomes for students with significant disabilities during their last year in public school (i.e., typically age 21): individualized and integrated direct-hire employment, postsecondary education, and access to a wide range of preferred community activities and environments. This model utilized a one-stop workforce investment strategy (Workforce Investment Act [WIA] of 1998, PL 105-220) that unified the three primary systems responsible through enabling legislation for this transition. It resulted in students exiting school with a stable paid job and a scheduled routine for obtaining nonwork activities in natural community environments when they were not working, and it ensured the continued support (often intensive and ongoing) needed to maintain these activities after graduation.

Model Implementation Prior to Graduation

This system unification was accomplished in two stages. The first stage occurred prior to exit from school; the second stage was implemented after exit. First, during participating students' last year in public school, the school system entered into a formal service arrangement with a private nonprofit agency that agreed to work with pending graduates before and after graduation. This agency was referred to as a *hybrid agency* because it was vendorized as a provider by both the rehabilitation and developmental disability systems, and was prepared to provide the services and supports needed to totally immerse students with significant disabilities in work and nonwork activities prior to graduation. Given the fact that these students were too old to attend a public high school (i.e., typically 21 years old), and did not wish to be enrolled full-time in community college or other postsecondary classes, this total community immersion approach eliminated the need to assign these students to a fixed classroom or school site. As a result, all of their instruction took place in natural community environments where the skills being acquired were functional and age-appropriate.

The participating school system shared the responsibility for developing preferred work and nonwork activities for the pending graduates with their designated hybrid nonprofit agency. In the majority of the demonstration sites, the school district dedicated a teacher to these students but subcontracted funds to the hybrid agency to provide the equivalent of instructional aides, thus redirecting existing staffing funds generated by the instructional student load. As a result, instruction and support were provided for a student's entire last year under school responsibility by both the teacher and hybrid agency staff prior to graduation. This established a formal link for students and their families with the hybrid agency and gave them a full academic year to evaluate the appropriateness of the agency and its services prior to exit. Entry into the TSIM during a student's last year in school was voluntary and at the discretion of the student and his or her family. If the pending graduate and his or her family were not satisfied with this approach to adult life, they were free to choose any other provider funded by either the rehabilitation or developmental disability system after they exited public school (or they could request a change of school placement prior to graduation).

In addition, the teacher typically shared office space at the hybrid agency so that all services and scheduling were planned jointly by the teacher, subcontracted agency support staff, and the agency's director. As a result, the hybrid agency became intimately familiar with each student's needs and skills and had the opportunity to gain insights from the teacher. This close collaboration for an entire school year enabled the hybrid agency to be more prepared to maintain and expand support for these students after graduation, using the same staff that had been involved prior to graduation. By the time the student exited school, the hybrid agency intimately understood the individual's support needs and interests, and the individual with significant disabilities and his or her family already had an established relationship with the provider.

Model Implementation After Graduation

During the participating students' last year in school, a formal policy management group was formed at each demonstration site, comprised of representatives from the public school system, rehabilitation system, and DDS. These management groups met on a regular basis to discuss student progress in both work and nonwork areas and to resolve policy or service issues. The management groups included system representatives with administrative decision-making authority, as well as direct services staff. Consistent with the approach described in the WIA, this meeting process was used as the formal single point of entry for requesting authorization for the continuation of services by the hybrid agency from the rehabilitation and developmental disabilities systems following graduation. As such, this hybrid agency functioned as a sole source for referral for these pending graduates, predicated on the informed choice of the students. Furthermore, for those systems that engaged in this model for multiple years, this meeting structure not only allowed for review of new student participants but also enabled review of the continued progress of graduates, providing a reliable source of information on long-term success.

A nuance in the provision of services for adults with significant disabilities that was developed through this model involved securing authorization from the rehabilitation system and DDS to fund support concurrently for the same individual. Prior to the implementation of this model in most regional jurisdictions in California, if the rehabilitation system was providing service for an individual, DDS would not provide services until support from the rehabilitation system was terminated. Likewise, the opposite prevailed if a graduate first obtained services after graduation from DDS. As a result, a student was faced with an untenable dilemma at the point of transition from public school. He or she 1) could seek a rehabilitation-funded supported employment program and secure employment assistance but have no support for nonwork needs or 2) seek a developmental disability–funded provider and have support for nonwork needs, yet postpone or forego employment. We view such categorical fragmentation of an individual's needs for service as counter-productive, counter-intuitive, and centered on the system, not the individual.

Through our model implementation efforts, we were successful in negotiating with the rehabilitation system and DDS to pay simultaneously for services for the same individual without falling victim to perceived problems of "double payment." This change in policy was accomplished simply by splitting the funding responsibility within the mandated parameters of each system. As such, the rehabilitation system authorized and provided all support needed for employment, while DDS authorized and provided support for all nonwork activities. The private nonprofit agency receiving this simultaneous funding from both systems was referred to as a hybrid agency to distinguish it from single-system providers. This dual-system funding maintained the holistic services that the public school system provided prior to graduation and eliminated the need to obtain the services of multiple agencies following graduation in order to meet all of an individual's support needs.

Accomplishments and Outcomes

The TSIM has been piloted successfully by us in metropolitan San Francisco, San Diego, and seven other selected communities in California, with more communities inquiring about the process. In addition, a first step was taken to broaden the national impact of this model through an agreement for model implementation in Montgomery County, Maryland. Beginning in September 2000, a 3-year plan was designed to expand the model throughout that state supported partially by federal demonstration funding.

Although the total number of students served is small in comparison to the number of students with disabilities exiting the school system, the approach is producing positive outcomes. In the first 3 years of implementation in the participating 11 school districts, 75% of the students were employed at graduation. About 91% of these students made the transition seamlessly to the same hybrid agency that had worked with them prior to graduation (Pumpian, Certo, & Sax, 1999), that is, with no disruption in services. On average, the hourly wage ($6.05) exceeded minimum wage and employees worked an average of 14.4 hours each week. Nearly all graduates left school with well-developed schedules of preferred nonwork activities in place, including recreation, leisure, and postsecondary courses. They also had transportation skills or support in place to maintain these activities.

The largest school district that has participated in the model identified 12 of the exiting students the first year of the project. Three years later, this became the new way of doing business. The district served all 44 of its exiting students identified with significant disabilities. The district began a partnership with one agency, subcontracting with the agency to provide services for the 12 students. With the number of exiting students increasing each year, within 2 years the original agency was no longer able to meet the needs of all the students. The following year, the district expanded the partnership to four agencies via subcontracts. The transition teacher and his staff, with input from the agency staff, administrators, students, and families, identified a list of criteria by which to match each student with one of the agencies. These included where the student lived, job interests, transportation issues, personal care needs, and other interests. Almost all of the matches were successful, and a spirit of collaboration among the agencies emerged as the staff shared effective strategies and faced similar challenges (Sax, 2000).

Implications of the Model

As discussed previously, prior to graduation each new hybrid agency participated actively with public school staff in a youth-centered decision-making process for career and community skill selection. This resulted in seamless continuation and new services for these same students, supported by the rehabilitation and developmental disabilities systems after they exited from the local schools. Based on our current experience in California, this arrangement significantly minimized the disruption typically experienced when making a transition of services across service systems (Certo et al., 1997; Gerry & Certo, 1992). The costs of these postschool employment, career enhancement, postsecondary education, and community living services were split differentially between two systems (rehabilitation and developmental disabilities) with rehabilitation being responsible for work support and developmental disabilities being responsible for support of nonwork activities.

Due to the mandates of the WIA and the Ticket to Work and Work Incentive Improvement Act of 1999 (PL 106-170), we anticipate that the number of participating systems providing services through the TSIM should expand over the next several years of implementation. In fact, an interagency agreement between the California Department of Rehabilitation and the California Department of Education was signed in August 2000 to publicly announce the intended collaboration between the departments to better meet the needs of students with disabilities entering the adult services system. A series of cross-agency trainings were funded to help increase awareness and provide opportunities for staff to develop strategies, such as those implemented through the TSIM.

Community Activities During Off-Work Hours

Another outgrowth of the model relates to supporting individuals with significant disabilities whose needs extend beyond employment and, therefore, cut across the perceived "boundaries" of rehabilitation and developmental disabilities. By design, TSIM has taken a broader view of collaboration and brought it to a new level where resources and responsibility for the same students at the same point in time have been shared jointly within the minimal regulatory constraints of each system. Because most individuals with significant disabilities who work do so part time (Wehman, 2001), significant portions of each day remain where support is needed for obtaining normalized community activities during off-work hours, such as recreation, postsecondary education, use of stores and services, and living arrangements. Although supporting such activities during off-work hours is permitted under certain circumstances within the Vocational Rehabilitation Act Amendments of 1943, state Departments of Rehabilitation have no clear mandate for providing such services; however, the state departments of developmental disabilities do, making cost sharing within a one-stop framework a logical alternative for the provision of holistic services.

Capacity Building

Through our efforts in California we have found that, collectively, the three participating systems have sufficient funds to pay for the direct services needed to develop careers and related community living skills. The critical pieces that were missing were a cadre of hybrid agencies or programs established to provide leadership for local communities through the TSIM and encouragement and support for the expansion of the TSIM across other providers. We have found that once these hybrid agencies were in place and the initial demonstration of the services, outcomes, and funding configuration was successful and standardized, additional local programs willingly joined their ranks. Their reasons for joining included the following: 1) the leadership example they provided encouraged other agencies to participate; 2) the model changed the pattern of referral for graduates, so local agencies needed to participate in order to continue to receive referrals; and 3) the operating costs tended to be the same or only slightly higher. Finally, through joint participation and an analysis of service needs, the postschool systems, most notably, the California Department of Rehabilitation, have been able to share some direct services costs with public schools prior to graduation, adding to the incentives for hybrid agencies to participate.

As the model expands throughout California and Maryland, we can begin to test the ability to generalize the model to other states. We believe that the configuration of this service delivery model and the information we have learned through its implementation have improved the process of transition from school to adulthood for individuals with significant disabilities, resulting in better outcomes and the promise of a more inclusive adult lifestyle for these graduates. Let's return to Jaime to see how his transition might have occurred under the TSIM model.

A NEW WAY FOR JAIME

After more training, Jaime was hired part time, subsidized by state funding that reimbursed the employer for a percentage of his wages. Now that Jaime was able to continue his work at the grocery store, rather than give up the work as is typically the case with a rotational job sampling site, additional adaptations and modifications were identified. These helped to increase Jamie's endurance and enhance his ability to learn more jobs in the store, increasing his overall independence. For example, his time card was color coded, making it easier to for him to find it and punch in. He continued to refer to his picture lists and store diagrams as necessary, and he also used a plastic guide for "fronting" items on the shelves, that is, bringing items to the front of the shelf for better visibility. He seemed to have a real knack for maintaining the produce bins and was learning how and when to water certain items as well as how to code the produce with stickers. He used a reacher with a customized rubber gripper on the end to turn the water on and off and had all sorts of unique holsters that attached to his wheelchair to hold the tools he used most often. Jaime's family was very pleased with his success and felt some relief in knowing that Jaime's immediate employment future was secure. By the time Jaime turned 21 in the fall of his "point of transition" year, he decided to apply for a permanent job in the grocery store and requested an interview with the manager. The interview went smoothly, and Jaime was hired to work 15 hours per week.

All the years of person-centered planning and futures mapping meetings paid off. Jaime and his family were introduced to staff from one of the agencies that was subcontracted with his school district to pave the way for Jaime's seamless transition. A meeting was held early that fall that included Jaime, his parents, his DDS case manager, his transition teacher, a rehabilitation counselor, and agency staff. Jaime's DDS file had been reactivated the prior spring, just to alert everyone to the impending changes. He also applied to the Department of Rehabilitation to open a case. A counselor from the Department of Rehabilitation agreed to come up with funding in October to fund the supports that Jaime needed on his job.

As his hours and responsibilities increased, new issues arose that required teaching Jaime some new skills and how to use unfamiliar equipment. His work hours increased to 20 hours a week and included time outside the school day. Transportation became a bigger issue, but the public bus system was available on most days, and his family pitched in on the others. The agency staff person insisted that Jaime take part in the problem solving, a skill that Jaime was eager to learn. Jaime's teacher continued to work with him on identifying courses he wanted to take in the local community college and exploring other community activities that he could join in his neighborhood.

All went smoothly, and by the end of the first semester, Jaime and his family decided to stay with the agency. The same agency support person would continue to work with Jaime after exiting the following summer. A seamless transition was in sight with the first day out of school looking essentially no different than his last day in school. Jaime had a job, a membership at the Young Men's Christian Association so he could swim, involvement in his Neighborhood Watch committee, and plans for attending a computer class at the community college. Now if he could just find a girlfriend!

REFERENCES

Affleck, J.Q., Edgar, E., Levine, P., & Kortering, L. (1990). Postschool status of students classified as mentally retarded, learning disabled, or nonhandicapped: Does it get better with time? *Education and Training in Mental Retardation, 25,* 315–324.

Blackorby, J., & Wagner, M. (1996). Longitudinal post school outcomes of youth with disabilities: Findings from the national longitudinal transition study. *Exceptional Children, 62,* 399–413.

Bush, G.W. (2001). *Executive summary: Fulfilling America's promise to Americans with disabilities* (Available: http://www.whitehouse.gov/news/freedominitiative/freedominitiative.html)

Butterworth, J., & Gilmore, D. (2000, June–July). Are we there yet?: Trends in employment opportunities and supports. *TASH Newsletter, 26,* 5–7.

Certo, N.J., Pumpian, I., Fisher, D., Storey, K., & Smalley, K. (1997). Focusing on the point of transition. *Education and Treatment of Children, 20*(1), 68–84.

Fisher, D., Sax, C., & Pumpian, I. (1999). *Inclusive high schools: Learning from contemporary classrooms.* Baltimore: Paul H. Brookes Publishing Co.

Gerry, M.H., & Certo, N.J. (1992). Current activity at the federal level and the need for service integration. *The Future of Children, 2*(1), 118–126.

Individuals with Disabilities Education Act (IDEA) Amendments of 1997, PL 105-17, 20 U.S.C. §§ 1400 *et seq.*

Individuals with Disabilities Education Act (IDEA) of 1990, PL 101-476, 20 U.S.C. §§ 1400 *et seq.*

Kohler, P.D., & Hood, L.K. (2000). *Improving student outcomes: Promising practices and programs for 1999–2000. A directory of innovative approaches for providing transition services for youth with disabilities.* Champaign, IL: Transition Research Institute, University of Illinois.

La Plante, M.P., Kennedy, J., Kaye, H.S., & Wenger, B.L. (1996). Disability and employment. *Disability statistics abstract, No. 11.* Washington, DC: U.S. Department of Education, National Institute on Disability and Rehabilitation Research: 1–4.

Lanterman Developmental Disabilities Services Act, Stats. 1976, Ch. 1252.

Mank, D. (1994). The underachievement of supported employment: A call for reinvestment. *Journal of Disability Policy Studies, 5,* 1–24.

McGaughey, M.J., Kiernan, W.E., McNally, L.C., & Gilmore, D.S. (1995). A peaceful coexistence?: State MR/DD agency trends in integrated employment and facility-based services. *Mental Retardation, 33*(3), 170–180.

National Council on Disability (NCD)/Social Security Administration (SSA) (November 1, 2000). *Transition and post-school outcomes for youth with disabilities: Closing the gaps to post-secondary education and employment.* (Available: http://www.ncd.gov/newsroom/publications/transition_11–1-00.html#1)

Pumpian, I., & Certo, N.J. (1996–1999). *Focusing on the point of transition: A service integration model.* Funded by U.S. Department of Education, Office of Special Education Programs, Postsecondary Model Demonstration Program, Washington, DC.

Pumpian, I., Certo, N.J., & Sax, C. (1999). *Progress Report, Year 02, AY 97–98: Focusing on the point of transition: A service integration model.* Funded by U.S. Department of Education, Office of Special Education Programs, Postsecondary Model Demonstration Program, Washington, DC.

Pumpian, I., Fisher, D., Certo, N.J., & Smalley, K. (1997). Changing jobs: An essential part of career development. *Mental Retardation, 35*(1), 39–48.

Rehabilitation Act Amendments of 1992, PL 102-569, 29 U.S.C. §§ 701 *et seq.*

Sax, C. (2000). Do systems really change? The point of transition service integration project. *TASH 1999 Conference Yearbook, 1*(1), 163–169.

School-to-Work Opportunities Act of 1994, PL 103-239, 20 U.S.C. §§ 6101 *et seq.*

Szymanski, E.M., Hanley-Maxwell, C., & Asselin, S.B. (1992). Systems interface: Vocational rehabilitation, special education, and vocational education. In F.R. Rusch, L. DeStefano, J. Chadsey-Rusch, L.A. Phelps, & E. Szymanski (Eds.), *Transition from school to adult life: Models, linkages, and policy* (pp. 153–171). Sycamore, IL: Sycamore.

Ticket to Work and Work Incentive Improvement Act (TWWIIA) of 1999, PL 106-170, 42 U.S.C. §§ 1305 *et seq.*

U.S. Bureau of the Census. (1992). *Labor force status and other characteristics of persons with a work disability.* Washington, DC: Author.

Vocational Rehabilitation Act Amendments of 1943, Ch. 190, 57 Stat. 374. 29 U.S.C. §§ 3141 *et seq.*

Wagner, M., & Blackorby, J. (1996). Transition from high school to work or college: How special education students fare. *The Future of Children, 6*(1), 103–120.

Wehman, P. (2001). *Life beyond the classroom: Transition strategies for young people with disabilities* (3rd ed.). Baltimore: Paul H. Brookes Publishing Co.

Wehman, P., Revell, G., & Kregel, J. (1997). Supported employment: A decade of rapid growth and impact. In P. Wehman & J. Kregel (Eds.), *Supported employment research: Expanding competitive employment opportunities for persons with significant disabilities.* Richmond, VA: Virginia Commonwealth University–Rehabilitation Research and Training Center.

Wehman, P., & West, M. (1996). Expanding supported employment opportunities for persons with severe disabilities. *TASH Newsletter, 22*(6), 24–27.

Wehman, P., West, M., Kregel, J., & Kane-Johnson, K. (1997). *Improving access to competitive employment for persons with developmental disabilities as a means of reducing social security expenditures.* Richmond, VA: Virginia Commonwealth University–Rehabilitation Research and Training Center. (Available: http://www.worksupport.com/Archives/improvingaccess.asp)

Workforce Investment Act of 1998, PL 105-220, 29 U.S.C. §§ 794d.

10

Putting Transition Plans into Action
"I Don't Want to Count Money at Home Anymore!"

Caren L. Sax and Colleen A. Thoma

FACING ANN'S FUTURE

Ann was 17 years old before she and her family seriously began a formal, coordinated transition assessment and planning process. Although transitions had occurred throughout Ann's life—from preschool into kindergarten, elementary to middle school, self-contained classroom to an inclusive classroom in her neighborhood school, and middle to high school—this was the BIG TRANSITION! It seemed as if the family had always helped Ann to think about her future, but the reality of this looming passage finally hit as Ann's peers began talking about applying to college. Major changes were not so far away. Ann had some definite ideas early on about her life as an adult that were revisited as she neared her 22nd birthday. She initially wanted a white Jeep, a family of her own, and a job. After acquiring her first job, her dreams expanded to finding an apartment with a roommate, getting a job where she could help others, and pursuing travel opportunities. Ann still hoped to own a Jeep, get married, and maybe have a child, but she added new dreams and goals as a result of further assessment, new experiences, and a newly developed sense of self-determination. She learned to set goals for herself with help, support, and encouragement from others who cared about her.

Ann's mom and dad, Edie and Bob, were and continued to be her greatest supporters and sources of confidence and strength. Edie said that planning for Ann's future was much like planning for the futures of her other two daughters, both of whom were older than Ann. "We want the same kinds of things for her that we want for our other daughters; we want them to have a job they enjoy, someone who cares about them, and enough time and money to live a comfortable life. Our goals for all three girls are the same, but we're finding that the steps to help them get there are different. They each need the right tools and preparation, as well as our support. For Ann, we're still discovering what the right tools and preparation might be, and the transition assessment process has played an important role."

PUTTING IT TOGETHER

Wise transition assessment requires more than one key meeting among students, families, professionals, and related services providers to complete the mandated program plans. Transition assessment, just like transition planning, is a continual process that helps students and their families make thoughtful and wise choices for a quality adult life. This book has described the philosophy and values that underpin wise transition assessment and has provided tools and strategies that can be useful for students and other stakeholders as they face changes in students' lives. A wealth of information can be generated from formal, informal, alternative, and other creative assessments; however, little of it will be useful if an action plan is not designed, implemented, and revisited on a regular basis. Likewise, little of this information will be useful unless action plans reflect student choices and honor family dynamics.

In this final chapter, the story of Ann and her family as they experienced Ann's transition from school to adult life illustrates the way in which information gathered from a variety of assessment procedures translates into specific actions that lead to an easier entry into adult life. The keys to wise transition planning are highlighted throughout the story, concluding with the themes and corresponding actions that must be implemented by all the important players.

MAKING ACTION PLANS

The first formal step in Ann's transition assessment and planning process involved a futures planning meeting, or Making Action Plans (MAPS; Forest & Lusthaus, 1990). Ann's teacher learned about this *person-centered planning process* in one of her graduate courses. Ironically, Ann's mother learned about this process at a conference during the same time frame. MAPS was presented as a strategy for helping families and professionals create a common vision for someone's future. That's exactly what the process did for Ann and her parents.

"It put transition and Ann's future into the whole educational planning process," her mother said. "It was the first time, I think, that the school personnel looked at more than just Ann's education. They had to look at her whole life and make sure that plans and goals fit into the big picture. It provided a whole new level of accountability."

The planning process became a primary source of transition assessment information. Ann had control of the guest list. She invited one of her friends, a friend of the family, a woman who worked with Ann after school, a few school personnel, and, of course, her parents. Everyone shared hopes and dreams as well as their fears. For example, Bob feared that Ann might forget to turn off a burner and start a fire if she lived alone. Edie feared that Ann might be victimized because of her trusting and outgoing nature that led her to converse with almost everyone she met. The family friend feared that Ann would be lost in the maze of human services where control by others and limited options were the norm. Recognizing and discussing these fears led to thinking about and planning for Ann's future goals in some new ways. During the individualized education program (IEP) meeting held the following week, Ann's plans addressed these long-range goals:

1. Provide in-home safety instruction for Ann so that she could learn the skills required to operate appliances safely and effectively, and involve her father in helping to assess her progress.

2. Teach Ann to use public transportation, with additional instruction and practice for initiating appropriate and safe social interactions.

3. Investigate adult services agencies to determine their philosophy, mission, values, and practices.

Another important part of the transition assessment process for Ann was the use of *alternative, performance-based assessments*. These methods provided opportunities for her to identify interests and preferences by experiencing specific activities in real environments, such as jobsites and postsecondary education environments. Ann's transition planning team used performance-based assessments to help Ann make decisions between options that were hard to explain or that were beyond Ann's ability to clearly visualize. For example, she did not understand the difference between attending postsecondary education for academic credit versus attending continuing education classes for personal enrichment. She was also confused about the distinction between attending community college and a 4-year university.

In order to learn more about these issues, Ann enrolled in a pilot course at the local community college that was designed for high school students who were considering college. This course introduced students to the expectations that exist at college, including exposure to the amount of reading required, different test formats (e.g., multiple-choice tests using computer forms, timed tests, short-answer quizzes, essay tests), and the range of teaching styles. They explored campus resources (e.g., library, tutoring, financial aid, health services, services for students with disabilities) and visited classes to observe first-hand the ways in which students and teachers interacted. As a result of participating in this experience, Ann decided to enroll in courses typically offered for continuing education. She was more interested in special interest adult education courses such as cake decorating, cooking, and other hobbies than in enrolling in courses for academic credit, at least as a first step. Such hands-on experiences, or *authentic assessments*, provide opportunities for students to make wise and thoughtful decisions about their lives based on real world experiences.

The focus on *self-determination* was essential for the success of Ann's transition assessment and planning process. The person-centered planning process inspired the school-based stakeholders to listen to Ann's ideas for the future and not make decisions for her. Ann and her mother saved the notes from her original MAPS meeting and the annual and short-term goals in a computer file. This made it easier for Ann and her family to review these goals, record progress, and make decisions about necessary changes. Having all the information in one place made the efforts more convenient and the actions more consistent. Too often, professionals who are not personally familiar with conducting an in-depth person-centered planning process may conclude that this approach is too time-consuming to implement with all their constituents. Edie refuted this assumption and explained the positive aspects of using this approach.

"I wish that teachers and other stakeholders who think that these meetings and approaches are too time-consuming would just try it!" Edie said. "If they could only see that if you put that effort in at the beginning, it makes the job easier in the long run. It really has been worth it for us. You don't just do it because you learned this new tool or new approach and you're using it for the sake of using the tool; you do it because it works . . . and makes the whole process more meaningful."

Edie also shared the importance of not only teaching self-determination skills to students with disabilities but also teaching the other stakeholders in the process to listen to, and really hear, the students who voice their preferences. After graduating from high school, Ann worked at a local restaurant where her hours and responsibilities increased as she built skills, confidence, and endurance. She also had a community support assistant who taught skills that Ann would need to live in her own apartment. Her school transition IEP and individualized transition plan (ITP) meetings were replaced by individualized service plan (ISP) meetings. Ann continued to use the list of goals that her mother helped her to keep updated on the computer.

During the first of her ISP meetings, the members of the team noticed that Ann had this list of goals and asked her to start the discussion by sharing her ideas and preferences. This was a good beginning to the meeting; however, some of the professionals seemed to struggle with truly hearing what Ann had to say and not reacting to her requests in traditional, systems-based ways. For example, one of the goals that Ann wanted to address was to improve her ability to use money, particularly at the grocery store. Although she had some basic skills, she still felt somewhat uncomfortable and wanted to increase her proficiency and confidence. Her community support assistant had worked with Ann to improve her ability to count money while at home and believed that this should be a continuing goal. Others at the meeting debated the importance of this goal for Ann, as Ann's standardized assessment data placed her at the moderate level of mental retardation.

These professionals typically recommended placing adults with that level of support needs in group homes and work enclaves. In these environments, a staff person would always be available to handle money for purchases. Edie and Ann reminded the team members that Ann's plans were to assume more control in her own life and that she wanted to go to a grocery store or other retail establishment independently. The team's next idea was to focus on having Ann count her change in her home, even though she already had the "next dollar" strategy in her repertoire. Ann became angry that her real goal was not heard and told the group emphatically, "I do not want to count money at home anymore!" To their credit, the group listened and changed the goal to reflect Ann's real preferences and needs (i.e., "Ann will use money to make purchases in the community"). More importantly, Ann set the tone for future meetings. Because of her skills in self-advocacy and self-determination, Ann's goals and preferences were heard and honored.

The process of helping Ann determine her *career/employment goals* utilized a variety of formal, informal, and alternate assessment methods. Of primary importance was providing opportunities to try jobs, using ecological inventories to determine the supports Ann needed to succeed at a particular job, as well as the natural resources available to provide those supports on an ongoing basis. Ann tried jobs at restaurants, nursing homes, child care centers, and her high school central office. Given the level of assistance that was necessary and the naturally occurring supports available at each location, the job at the restaurant was considered the best fit. After working there for a year and a half, Ann began providing natural support for other employees; that is, she often trained new employees on various jobs. Her new boss gave her even more responsibility, and Ann appeared to be thriving. She still had dreams of having a job that enabled her to teach self-advocacy skills and help other students with disabilities take control of their own transition planning process. She shared her story at local, state, and national conferences and started learning additional skills necessary to do more of this in the future. Ann added "speaking at more conferences" to her list of goals and dreams.

Although *traditional formal and curricular-based assessment* procedures did not play a major role in helping Ann make decisions about her life, they were an early part of the transition assessment process. Ann's school typically used the *Life Centered Career Education Curriculum* (Brolin, 1993) to help determine a student's abilities in a number of areas that are particularly important for transition planning. For example, in the area of cooking and daily living skills, Ann's assessment information indicated a need to teach her safety skills in the kitchen. This assessment information gave further impetus to Ann's goal to learn safety skills at home.

Ann, like most eighth graders who attend school in her state, was required to take a class on careers. Her teacher administered a variety of formal assessments, including interest inventories and aptitude tests. These formal assessments gave Ann a place to start her career exploration process, narrowing down the career fields to service and health care. More focused time and energy was then placed on job shadowing, ecological inventories, and other authentic assessments to provide supporting information about the appropriateness of specific job opportunities.

WISE PRACTICES

What is clear from Ann's story, as well as the stories of the other students with disabilities shared throughout this book, is that the methods and strategies are just tools, and tools are only as good as those who use them. Every person-centered planning meeting has the potential of becoming yet another standardized procedure or program that, while going through the motions, does not necessarily integrate the philosophy and values essential to wise transition assessment and planning. If students must mold their goals to match the system's "slots" rather than the system creating services and supports to meet student needs, then ultimately, none of these strategies will make a difference. As Ann demonstrated, self-determination leads to self-advocacy. As a result, attitudes as well as actions of those representing the system can be changed.

All of the strategies, models, and ideas in this book have been presented with the following themes in mind. They bear repeating one more time, as we pursue wise transition assessment and planning.

1. *Respect the students as individuals.*
   - Listen to their ideas and hear their dreams.
   - Support them in making wise choices, and help them learn from the experience of making poor decisions.
   - Expose them to as many experiences as possible.
   - Identify what works as well as what does not work.
   - Hold high expectations and promote risk taking.
   - Accept it when they change their minds.

2. *Respect their families.*
   - Ask parents what they want for their sons and daughters.
   - Ask family members for their ideas.
   - Respect family dynamics and other influences.
   - Encourage families to dream.
   - Encourage them to dream big.
   - Listen to their fears and hear what it will take to ease them.
   - Accept it when families change their minds.

3. *Approach assessment and planning holistically.*
   - Appreciate the complexity of the individual.
   - Think about needs, interests, skills, preferences, and challenges—and how those might look in different environments.
   - Consider all possible supports and strategies—natural supports, reasonable accommodations, assistive technology, personal assistance, and creative uses of time, energy, materials, and other resources.
   - Recognize that everyone's future includes more than work and more than school and must include opportunities to build meaningful relationships.

4. *Work together as a team.*
   - Talk and listen as if you were planning your own future.
   - Build on the expertise of one another.

- Seek more information.
- Seek the correct information.
- Identify a common vision and mean it.
- Learn from one another.
- Check your values and expectations.
- Withhold judgment.
- Accept it when plans need to change.

Given the information and examples provided in this book, we hope that you can give *assessment* another chance. As we think about *assessment* in the original sense of the word, "to sit with," we believe that wise assessment practices can make the difference between maintaining the status quo for students with disabilities and their achieving a quality adult life. If we consider the broader functions of assessment—that is, not only assessing the individual, but also assessing the environment, activities, supports, and relationships that best match the needs of the individual—we are much more likely to see people with significant disabilities living life in the way that they want—with good friends and meaningful activities. Please keep this concept in mind as we close with a thought-provoking fable by Scot Danforth.

REFERENCES

Brolin, D.E. (1993). *The Life-Centered Career Education Curriculum.* Reston, VA: Council for Exceptional Children.

Forest, M., & Lusthaus, E. (1990). Everyone belongs with the MAPS action planning system. *Teaching Exceptional Children,* 22(2), 32–35.

Coda

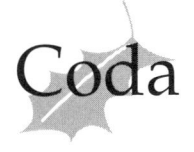

The Watergivers
A History of a Helping Profession

Scot Danforth

A FABLE FOR OUR TIMES

The first generation of Watergivers decided to place themselves at the very location of need itself. They stood at the edge of the vast and dry desert where many wandered in thirst. They stood there with jugs of cold water. Little by little, in dribs and drabs, the thirsty people of the desert came to the edge of the sand and quenched their thirst with the assistance of the Watergivers.

The second generation of Watergivers decided to improve on the work of the prior generation. They decided to sort the Desertwalkers into two groups, those deserving of water and those undeserving of water. Those deserving of water were persons who lacked means or ability to find, earn, or carry water on their own. The undeserving were persons who were fully able to work for water or find or carry their own water. These people were viewed as simply lazy or immoral. They came to the desert's edge for the easy, free water. The second generation of Watergivers decided to identify these undeserving Desertwalkers and refuse them water—for their own good.

This initial problem of sorting the Desertwalkers into the deserving and undeserving was soon further complicated. The third generation of Watergivers found that some Desertwalkers who came to drink the water remained thirsty despite drinking. No matter how much help the Watergivers gave, this specific group always wanted more. It seemed that their thirsts were unquenchable.

This third generation of Watergivers decided that watergiving was a complicated profession, so they gathered all the Watergivers for a big meeting. They formed a group called

The American Association for the Care of the Water Deficient and Chronically Thirsty (AACWDCT). The AACWDCT set four specific goals for their new professional group:

1. To develop scientific instruments for categorizing the Desertwalkers according to the following three classifications—1) deserving water-deficient; 2) undeserving water-deficient; and 3) chronic, incurably thirsty
2. To conduct basic research to understand the disease processes underlying water-deficiency and chronic thirst
3. To elevate the profession in the hearts and minds of the public
4. To provide information to the public about the disease of water-deficiency and chronic thirst so that the public could protect itself from the moral degradation and social disorder caused by those bearing these illnesses

To quote from the AACWDCT meeting record, "An association of professional men must rely on the scientific comprehension of problems burdening society in order to rightly develop programs to halt the social menace at hand and bring virtue to those in need of water."

The fourth generation of Watergivers built on this professional foundation, developing norm-referenced instruments to measure and categorize the many forms of diseased thirst. Many of the studies focused on two primary constructs: 1) water capacity (how much an individual can drink in a 90-minute session while observed by a qualified psychometrist holding a stopwatch) and 2) water retention (the extent to which one can hold one's water, thereby alleviating thirst). The latter construct led to the famous French water closet studies (later replicated in English at Stanford) in which water-deficient men were forced to drink a half-gallon of water and then spend 12 hours dancing from foot to foot outside a locked bathroom door.

The great achievement of the fourth generation was the standardization of diagnostic procedures for the various water-related disabilities and the bureaucratization of the watergiving process. By this point in history, the Watergivers had set up an elaborate maze at the edge of the desert, a system of channels and alleys that shuttled different types of water-deficients to different water service locations. The basic idea was that different types of water-deficients required different types of individualized beverage programs (IBPs): hard waters and soft waters, high-volume programs and low-volume programs, high-pressure delivery and low-pressure delivery, alternative beverages for those allergic to water, and thirst modification programs for those with chronic and incurable thirsts. Early records indicate that the Watergivers took great delight in seeing the innocent joy of a water-deficient imbibing and discharging water among his own kind, a safe and secluded environment where he could relax and live free of the social pressures of the main water stream.

Coda

The fifth generation of Watergivers were rabble-rousers and malcontents who decided that the location of beverage imbibement made a difference. They forged a path toward what they called "inclusive imbibement settings," opportunities for the water-deficient to drink at the mainstream trough with their nondeficient peers. This inclusive imbibement movement split the AACWDCT into antagonistic factions, those advocating for mainstream drinking for all and those who deemed such a social goal to be an unscientific "illusion."

The sixth generation of Watergivers decided to hold a meeting. One guy read a silly story about all sorts of nonsense. The Watergivers nodded and smiled politely so as to give him the impression that they went all the way to New Orleans to listen to a stupid story. Then, they decided to strip away the knowledge and ideas and practices built up by the many generations of Watergivers, to peel back all the layers of assumptions and truths and ideologies. The profession had built up a discourse and a jargon and a paternalism many layers thick, all resting on that first interpretation of the Desertwalkers' need and the Watergivers' role as helpers. Upon that first layer of need and help, they had built a thick science of deficiency, diagnosis, and treatment. They had built a notion of disease and created a profession for purposes of isolating and curing that disease.

The sixth generation looked at all these layers and decided to question everything. They questioned not only the professional construction of need but also all the scientific knowledge that had been built up and then assumed to be true, all the understandings eventually taken for granted about human deficiency and the profession that helps. They decided at that meeting to inquire critically in every way about everything.

BEYOND THE FABLE

I originally wrote this history of the development of a helping profession for a short speech I gave in April 2000 at the first meeting of the Disability Studies in Education (DSE) Special Interest Group of the American Education Research Association. I believe that we formed the DSE in order to bring to life the quest of the sixth generation, the need to question what had remained unquestioned in the various fields of disability service and research. But what should we question? And how will that help us serve students with disabilities during the transition years?

I'll start my look at what we should question by quoting the opening line of Joseph P. Shapiro's excellent history of the disability rights movement entitled *No Pity: People with Disabilities Forging a New Civil Rights Movement*: "Nondisabled Americans do not understand disabled ones" (1993, p. 3). This is a profound, sweeping, and stirring statement. It is especially disturbing to read this quotation at the close of a book on assessment, a book designed to help us understand and know students with disabilities in such a way that we can better support them. It seemed as if Shapiro was telling special education and rehabilitation professionals without disabilities to take a long hike off a short pier.

Not really—but close. Shapiro was simply a journalist who was passing on a message from the many Americans with disabilities he interviewed and hung around with in the process of writing his book. He was carrying a message from one side of the (dis)ability wall to the other, from disability culture to nondisability culture. Americans with disabilities told him in so many ways: Folks without disabilities don't know what it is like to be me, to be in this body, to be in this mind. They do not know the experience of having a disability. They know only what it is like to be a person without a disability who thinks about what it might be like to have a disability. So, they view us in terms of how we fall short of what they think we ought to be. They can't know what it is like to simply be the person whom others think is falling short.

This message is difficult for Americans without disabilities to hear, but those who are open and compassionate about human differences are able to fathom this message. We have heard and hopefully learned from similar messages from other minority groups in recent decades. We have learned from the women's movement that the experience of being a woman is beyond the understanding and words of men. We have learned similar lessons in relation to race and ethnicity. To those within the American public who have been paying attention to the development of many political identities in recent decades, the quote from Shapiro is another version of a lesson we have learned before.

But special educators and other professionals who work closely every day with individuals with disabilities often have difficulty hearing Shapiro's lesson. We might wonder how we could *not* understand Americans with disabilities and still call ourselves qualified professionals.

Special education teachers might say, "If anyone knows these students and knows what their lives are like, it is me. I spend 30 hours a week with kids with disabilities. I've been doing this work for 15 years. How can anyone say that I don't understand my students?"

Disability researchers might say, "Of course, there is always much more for us to know, but we have done decades of excellent research on various types of disabilities. We have a strong understanding of what causes these disabilities and how these disabilities impact the lives of children and their families. We have a pretty good understanding of the kinds of interventions that work to help these families. But we can always know more. The science is good, but it can get better. We must rededicate ourselves to our research in order to discover more in the future."

In the story of the Watergivers, I told about how the profession grew in legitimacy and influence within society as the profession claimed a greater and more scientific knowledge base. In the development of the helping professions like special education, psychology, psychiatry, and social work, this growth of legitimacy and a scientific (or what was claimed as scientific) knowledge base about certain individuals or social problems occurred within the 20th century (see Jones, 1999; Trent, 1994). To sum it up neatly, becoming a real profession and a real professional in modern America has required that the professionals claim to know more and better about the clientele they are serving than the clientele know about themselves. The standard cultural story about the progress of social science tells us that research will continue to move professionals closer and closer to the truth. In addition, we tell ourselves that our act of moving closer and closer to the truth is for the good of the clientele we serve.

Now we step back again and think about the message that Shapiro brought to Americans without disabilities from those with disabilities. We special educators are stuck in a difficult quandary. On the one hand, we are supposed to hold a greater knowledge about disabilities than people who have disabilities and their family members. Our field has relied on that greater, scientific knowledge as the source of our legitimacy. We are typically taught that knowledge in our university professional education. If not for that greater knowledge, what kind of professionals are we? What kind of profession is this if we do not know better than the nonprofessionals?

But also, if we hear the message carried by Shapiro and allow it to run deep enough within us that we begin to question, then we're back to the issue of what to question. To me, in my reading of Shapiro (1993) and in my listening to rich literature now coming forth from persons with disabilities (e.g., Russell, 1998; Charlton, 1998) who are patient enough to offer guidance to special educators and other professionals, the message is this: "Question your need and desire to know and understand a person with a disability in a way that you consider superior to that individual's understanding of him- or herself. Question that need deeply enough, firmly enough, often enough, that you hear yourself less and you will hear that individual more. In the case of an individual who does not communicate verbally (even with many modes of augmentative and alternative communication), you can listen to that individual's nonverbal language, listen to the language of that person's life story until you learn to hear in the nonverbal language that the person is using. And you can listen to family members and loved ones who know this person through the bonds of intimacy, friendship, and commitment."

The challenge to the present generation of Watergivers is to question all we think we know. If we question deeply and fully enough, we may learn to listen to those we assumed we understood. Then, we will find ourselves back at the beginning of our history, at the very location of need itself. Except this time, we will be at the location of need as defined by those we serve rather than as defined by the traditions and knowledge base of our profession.

REFERENCES

Charlton, J.I. (1998). *Nothing about us without us: Disability oppression and empowerment.* Berkeley: University of California Press.

Jones, K.W. (1999). *Taming the troublesome child: American families, child guidance, and the limits of psychiatric authority.* Cambridge, MA: Harvard University Press.

Russell, M. (1998). *Beyond ramps: Disability at the end of the social contract: A warning from an uppity crip.* Monroe, ME: Common Courage Press.

Shapiro, J.P. (1993). *No pity: People with disabilities forging a new civil rights movement.* New York: Times Books.

Trent, J.W. (1994). *Inventing the feeble mind: A history of mental retardation in the United States.* Berkeley: University of California Press.

Index

Page numbers followed by "*f*" indicate figures; those followed by "*t*" indicate tables.

Abandonment, of assistive technology (AT), 89–90
Action plans, *see* Person-centered planning
ADA, *see* Americans with Disabilities Act (ADA) of 1990 (PL 101-336)
Agency-directed services, 14–15
Alternative assessments
   backward design process, 82–84, 84*t*
   case study, 71–72, 135
   characteristics of, 74
   definitions of
      authentic assessment, 76–77
      demonstration of mastery, 78
      discourse assessment, 78
      formative/summative assessment, 77
      performance assessment, 76
      performance tasks, 79
      portfolio, 77
      profile, 78–79
      project work, 78
      simulation, 79–80
   scoring methods for
      assessment lists, 81
      checklists, 80–81
      rubrics, 80
      score cards, 81
      student self-evaluation, 81–82
   versus traditional assessments, 72–74, 75–76*t*
   in vocational/career development, 107–108, 108*t*
American Institute of Research Self-Determination Scale, 31
Americans with Disabilities Act (ADA) of 1990 (PL 101-336), 88
Arc's Self-Determination Scale, The, 30–31
Artificial environments, 54, 105
Assessment
   alternative approaches
      backward design process, 82–83, 84*t*
      case study, 71–72
      characteristics of, 74
      definitions of, 76–80
      scoring methods, 80–82
      versus traditional, 72–74, 75–76*t*
   case study, 1–2

147

Assessment—continued
  definition of, 2
  formal approaches, 26, 30–31, 52
  informal approaches
    case study, 51
    examples of, 26, 52, 57
    proposed model
      assumptions of, 52–54
      descriptive application of, 64–66
      eight steps of, 54–64, 55*t*
      strength of, 52
      summary of, 66
  overarching questions, 9–10
  person-centered approaches, 14, 15–19, 21, 134–137
  purpose for, 8–9, 54–56, 64
  in self-determination
    assessing interests and preferences, 27–29
    case study, 25–26
    curricular and program resources, 32–36
    determining instructional needs, 29–31
    promoting student involvement, 31–32
    summary, 36
    using multiple approaches, 26–27
  in vocational/career development, 107–108, 108*t*
  wise practices for, 137–139
  see also specific assessments
Assessment lists, 81
Assistive technology (AT), 87–100
  case study, 87
  evaluation and selection of, 93–94
  importance of, 88–89
  Matching Person and Technology (MPT) evaluation process, 90–93, 96*f*, 97*f*, 100*t*
  reducing abandonment, 89–90
  STATEMENT project, 94–100, 99*t*
Assistive Technology Act of 1998 (PL 105-395), 88, 93
AT, *see* Assistive technology
Authentic assessment, 76–77, 135
Autonomous Functioning Checklist, 31

Behavioral observations, 57–58

Career development, *see* Vocational and career assessment
Career interest inventory, 114
Carl D. Perkins Vocational and Applied Technology Education Act Amendments of 1990 (PL 101-392), 104
CBI, *see* Community-based instruction
Central Remedial Clinic (CRC), 94
Checklists, 58, 80–81
ChoiceMaker Self-Determination Transition Assessment, 30
ChoiceMaker Self-Determination Transition Curriculum, 32, 33*t*
Choosing Goals lesson, 32
Client Technical Services (CTS), 94
Community sites, visitation etiquette for, 46–47
Community-based instruction (CBI), 6
Continuity for students, 42–46, 123
CRC, *see* Central Remedial Clinic
Criterion-referenced measures, 26, 114
CTS, *see* Client Technical Services
Cultural values, respecting, 53
Curriculum-based assessment, 26, 108*t*, 113–114, 137
Customized futures planning, 17–19, 18–19*f*

DDS, *see* Developmental disabilities service system
Demonstration of mastery, 78
Developmental disabilities service (DDS) system, 123, 125–126
Direct observation, 52, 57–58
Disabilities Studies in Education (DSE), 143
Disability profile, 94, 95*t*
Discourse assessment, 78
DO IT! problem-solving strategy, 33, 34*t*
Dropout rates for students with isabilities, 3
DSE, *see* Disabilities Studies in Education

Ecological inventory, 52, 61, 108*t*, 112, 112*t*
Education for All Handicapped Children Act of 1975 (PL 94-142), 3, 4, 32
Education system
  service delivery questions for

postsecondary years, 7–8
secondary years, 6–7
for students with disabilities
   effectiveness of, 3–4
   free appropriate public education, 41
   overview of opportunities in, 2–3
   segregated placements within, 4–6
Employment, *see* Vocational and career assessment
Employment sites, visitation etiquette for, 46–47
Empowerment evaluation, 29
Environmental assessments, 26, 46, 55, 56, 108*t*
Evaluation methods, 80–82
Event recording, 58, 59*f*
Exiting school, *see* Postschool outcomes

Fable about development of helping profession, 141–143
Family involvement in transition planning
  case study, 39–40
  collaboration and, 53
  constancy of, 47
  cultural values, 53
  support practices and strategies for
    conscientiousness of details, 46–47, 48*f*
    continuity for students, 42–46
    establishing credibility, 40–42
    unexpected challenges, 40
Feedback, effective, 82
Formal (standardized) assessment
  limited usefulness of, 52, 107–108
  in self-determination, 26, 30–31
  in vocational/career development, 107–108
Formative assessment, 77
Functional assessment, *see* Informal (functional) assessment
Futures planning meetings
  case study, 13, 133–134
  personalized themes and, 20–21, 22–23*f*
  person-centered process, 14, 15–19, 134–137
  values and, 21
  wise practices for, 137–139

Goal Action Planning, 36
Goals and objectives, prioritizing, 63, 66
Graduates, *see* Postschool outcomes

Hands-on experiences, *see* Authentic assessment
HEART, *see* Horizontal European Activities in Rehabilitation Technology report
Holistic services, 128
Home Inventory Form, 58
Horizontal European Activities in Rehabilitation Technology (HEART) report, 94, 98, 99*t*

I PLAN strategy, 35–36, 35*t*
IDEA, *see* Individuals with Disabilities Education Act Amendments of 1997 (PL 105-17); Individuals with Disabilities Education Act of 1990 (PL 101-476)
IEP, *see* Individualized education program
Inclusive education, emphasis on, 4–7, 15, 42, 122
Individualized education program (IEP), 43
  guide, 41
  individualizing, 14, 135
  least restrictive environment (LRE), 4–6
  legal processes and procedures, 41–42
  student involvement, 32, 60
Individualized service plan (ISP), 14, 136
Individualized transition plan (ITP), 14, 43, 136
Individuals with Disabilities Education Act (IDEA) Amendments of 1997 (PL 105-17), 3
  assessment components, 27, 57, 72
  assistive technology (AT) devices and services, 88
  least restrictive environment (LRE), 4–6
  parent participation rights, 41, 53
  passage of, 5
  postsecondary options, 121
  student participation rights, 33, 53
  vocational assessment components, 104
Individuals with Disabilities Education Act (IDEA) of 1990 (PL 101-476), 41, 72, 88

Informal (functional) assessment
  case study, 51
  conducting, 61, 63, 65
  examples of, 26, 52, 57
  proposed model
    assumptions of, 52–54
    descriptive application of, 64–66
    eight steps of, 54–64, 55*t*
  in self-determination, 30
  strength of, 52
  summary of, 66
  in vocational/career development, 107–108, 108*t*
Instructional needs, in self-determination
  assessment of, 29–31
  curricular and program resources, 32–36
  promoting student involvement, 31–32
Integration Quotient (IQ) questionnaire, 47, 48*f*
Interest inventory, 59–60, 108*t*, 114
  see also Preference assessment strategies
Interval recording, 58
Interviews, 26, 52, 58, 108*t*, 110–111
Inventories, *see* specific inventories
ISP, *see* Individualized service plan
ITP, *see* Individualized transition plan

Job analysis survey, 61
Job satisfaction, 115–116
Journals, used for self-assessment, 81–82

Kuder DD Occupational Interest Survey, 114

Lanterman Developmental Disabilities Services Act of 1976, 121
Laws, *see* Legislation
Learning style assessment, 26
Least restrictive environment (LRE) provision, 4–6, 41
Legislation, 4–5, 41, 104–105, 122
  see also specific laws
Life Centered Career Education Curriculum, 137
Longitudinal records, *see* Portfolio assessment
LRE, *see* Least restrictive environment provision

Making Action Plans (MAPS), 14, 17, 134–137
MAPS, *see* Making Action Plans
Mastery demonstration, 78
Matching Person and Technology (MPT)
  evaluation process, 90–93, 96*f*, 97*f*, 100*t*
Microswitches, 27
MPT, *see* Matching Person and Technology evaluation process
Multiple strategies, *see* Alternative assessments

Narrative recording, 57
Natural environments, 53–54
Neighborhood inventory, 111–112
Next S.T.E.P. (Student Transition and Educational Planning), 30, 34–35, 74, 77
Nonuse of assistive technology (AT), 89–90

Observations, informal, 26, 52, 57–58, 108*t*, 110
One-Stop Centers, 105
Outcomes, *see* Postschool outcomes

Parent rights, 41
  see also Individuals with Disabilities Education Act (IDEA) Amendments of 1997 (PL 105-17)
Participatory planning, emphasis on, 31–32
PATH, *see* Planing Alternative Tomorrows with Hope
Pennsylvania Association for Retarded Children v. Commonwealth of Pennsylvania (1971), 5
Performance tasks, 79
Performance-based assessment, 76, 82, 135
Personal futures planning, 14, 26
Person-centered planning
  versus agency-driven services, 14–15
  case study, 13, 133–134
  descriptive examples using, 15–19, 134–137
  personalized themes and, 20–21, 22–23*f*
  philosophy of, 14

qualitative study of, 15
values and, 21
vocational/career assessment and, 109
wise practices for, 137–139
Perspectives of others, obtaining, 56–57, 65
PL 93-112, *see* Rehabilitation Act of 1973
PL 94-142, *see* Education for All Handicapped Children Act of 1975
PL 100-407, *see* Technology Related Assistance for Individuals with Disabilities Act of 1988
PL 101-336, *see* Americans with Disabilities Act (ADA) of 1990
PL 101-392, *see* Carl D. Perkins Vocational and Applied Technology Education Act Amendments of 1990
PL 101-476, *see* Individuals with Disabilities Education Act (IDEA) of 1990
PL 102-569, *see* Rehabilitation Act Amendments of 1992
PL 103-239, *see* School-to-Work Opportunities Act of 1994
PL 105-17, *see* Individuals with Disabilities Education Act (IDEA) Amendments of 1997
PL 105-220, *see* Workforce Investment Act (WIA) of 1988
PL 105-394, *see* Assistive Technology Act of 1998
PL 106-170, *see* Ticket to Work and Work Incentive Improvement Act of 1999
Placement decisions, 4–6
Planning Alternative Tomorrows with Hope (PATH), 14, 20, 77
Planning meetings, *see* Futures planning meeting
Portfolio assessment
  avoiding pitfalls in, 45–46
  definition of, 77, 108t, 114
  essential components in, 44–45
Postschool outcomes
  assessment factors in, 116
  case study, 119–120
  critical issues in, 3–4, 120–122
  service delivery dilemmas, 122–124
    developmental disabilities service system (DDS), 123

rehabilitation system, 122–123
    special education system, 122
  Transition Service Integration Model (TSIM)
    accomplishments/outcomes of, 126–127
    case study, 129–130
    implementation efforts
      after graduation, 125–126
      prior to graduation, 124–125
    implications of, 127–129
Postsecondary education, emphasis on, 7–8, 121
Poverty rates, of students with disabilities, 121
Preference assessment strategies
  approach, 27
  expressive behavior, 28
  microswitch, 27
  observing responses over time, 29
  physical selection, 28
  task performance, 28
  time engagement, 28
Profiles, used to measure progress, 78–79, 108t, 109–110
Program assessment, 55–56
Projects, used to measure progress, 78
Purpose of assessment, 8–9, 54–56, 64

Quality of life, 2, 29–30
Questionnaires, 58, 108t, 110–111, 110t, 111t

Rehabilitation Act Amendments of 1992 (PL 102-569), 105, 121
Rehabilitation Act of 1973 (PL 93-112), 88
Rehabilitation system, 122–123
RESNA Technical Assistance Project, 93
Rubrics, used to measure progress, 80

Satisfaction, student, 115–116
School-to-Work Opportunities Act of 1994 (PL 103-239), 105, 121
Score cards, 81
Scoring methods, 80–82
Secondary education, emphasis on, 6–7
Segregated education, critique of, 4–7
Selection procedures, 57–61, 65

Self-Advocacy Strategy for Education and Transition Planning, 35–36
Self-assessment, 60, 81–82
Self-Determination: A Curriculum to Help Adolescents Learn to Achieve Their Goals, 30
Self-determined assessment
   case study, 25–26, 135–136
   components in
      curricular and program resources, 32–36
      determining instructional needs, 29–31
      promoting student involvement, 31–32
      students' interests and preferences, 27–29
   summary of, 36
   using multiple approaches, 26–27
Self-Directed IEP lessons, 32
Self-evaluation assessment, 29–31
Service delivery system
   dilemmas of, 122–124
   integration efforts of, 46–47, 48f
   questions about, 6–8
   unification model, 124–126
   see also Transition process
Severe disabilities, definition of, 4
Sheltered facilities, 105
Simulated environments, 54, 105
Simulation assessment, 79–80
Site visits, etiquette for, 46–47
Situational assessment, 26, 108t, 113
Social support assessment, 52, 60, 62f
Special education system, 122
Standardized tests, *see* Formal (standardized) assessment
STATEMENT, *see* Systematic Template for Assessing Technology Enabling Mainstream Education–National Trial project
Student involvement, 53
Student outcomes, *see* Postschool outcomes
Student self-evaluation, 60, 81–82
Student survey, 52, 58, 110t
Summative assessment, 77
Supported employment, 105
Surveys, 52, 58, 110–111, 110t, 111t

Systematic observation, 113
Systematic Template for Assessing Technology Enabling Mainstream Education–National Trial (STATEMENT) project, 94–100, 99t

Taking Action lessons, 32
Task analysis, 52, 58, 61, 63
Task-analytic rubrics, 80
Task performance, 28
Technical Assistance Alliance for Parent Centers, 41
Technology education skills assessment, 26
Technology-Related Assistance for Individuals with Disabilities Act of 1988 (PL 100-407), 93
Technology-related services, *see* Assistive technology (AT)
Ticket to Work and Work Incentive Improvement Act of 1999 (PL 106-170), 127
Time engagement strategy, 28
Traditional assessment
   reevaluation of, 72–74, 75–76t
   vocational/career evaluations and, 105–106
Transition process
   continuity for students, 42–46
   effective strategies, 44
   families and, 44
   legal processes and procedures, 41–42
   see also Postschool outcomes
Transition Service Integration Model (TSIM)
   accomplishments/outcomes of, 126–127
   case study, 129–130
   hybrid agency, 124
   implementation efforts
      after graduation, 125–126
      prior to graduation, 124–125
   implications of, 127–129
Transition Skills Inventory, 30, 34–35
TSIM, *see* Transition Service Integration Model

Unemployment statistics, 3, 121

Index

Values, family, 53
Verbal interview format, 111
Visiting worksites, etiquette for, 46–47
Vocational and career assessment
   case study, 103, 137
   concluding thoughts on, 116
   descriptive examples of, 107–108, 108*t*
      curriculum-based assessment, 113–114
      ecological inventory, 112, 112*t*
      interest inventory, 114
      interviews/questionnaires, 110–111, 110*t*, 111*t*
      neighborhood inventory, 111–112
      portfolios, 114
      situational assessment, 113
      workplace analysis, 112
   evaluating program effectiveness, 114–116
   general process of, 106–107
   guiding principles to, 106
   issues with traditional evaluations, 105–106
   legislation guiding, 104–105
   observations across environments, 110–113
   reform efforts in, 103–104
   visitation etiquette, 46–47
   vocational profiles, 109–110
Vocational profiles, 108*t*, 109–110
Vocational Rehabilitation Act Amendments of 1943, 128
Vocational/employability scale, 26

Whose Future Is It Anyway?: A Student-Directed Transition Planning Program, 32–34
WIA, *see* Workforce Investment Act of 1988
Work One Centers, 105
Workforce Investment Act (WIA) of 1988 (PL 105-220), 105, 124, 127
Workplace analysis, 112
Worksites, visitation etiquette for, 46–47